ADVANCED FUGITIVE

RUNNING, HIDING, SURVIVING AND *THRIVING* FOREVER

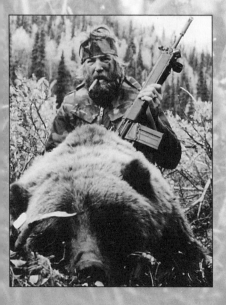

Kenn Abaygo

Paladin Press
Boulder, Colorado

Advanced Fugitive: Running, Hiding, Surviving and Thriving Forever
by Kenn Abaygo

Copyright © 1997 by Kenn Abaygo

ISBN 0-87364-933-8
Printed in the United States of America

Published by Paladin Press, a division of
Paladin Enterprises, Inc., P.O. Box 1307,
Boulder, Colorado 80306, USA.
(303) 443-7250

Direct inquiries and/or orders to the above address.

PALADIN, PALADIN PRESS, and the "horse head" design
are trademarks belonging to Paladin Enterprises and
registered in United States Patent and Trademark Office.

All rights reserved. Except for use in a review, no
portion of this book may be reproduced in any form
without the express written permission of the publisher.

Neither the author nor the publisher assumes
any responsibility for the use or misuse of
information contained in this book.

CONTENTS

	Introduction	1
1	The Fugitive's World: Here Be Dragons	5
2	Welcome Down Underground	15
3	Death from Afar: Avoiding and Countering the Sniper	29
4	Life on the Street: The Concrete Jungle	45
5	Primitive Prospects: The Wilderness Fugitive	69
6	All the Major Networks	103
7	Personal Weapons Selection	109
Appendix A	Firearms Training Sources	121
Appendix B	Survival Supply Sources	123
Appendix C	Firearms Accessory Supply Sources	127
Appendix D	Sources for Surveillance and Countersurveillance Devices	. . 129
Appendix E	Camouflage Clothing Sources	131
Appendix F	Survival Training Sources	135
Appendix G	Recommended Reading	137

For John L., an old Antarctica hand, SpecWar coxswain, Navy Seabee, and survivalist, whose skills few could equal. Gimme wisdom, John.

INTRODUCTION

"Could you feel your whole world fall apart and fade away?"

—Steely Dan
Kid Charlemagne

If push came to shove and you had to disappear for an extended period of time, intending either to come back to your old life eventually or start a new one, could you do it? Could you take all the steps necessary to survive for a year in the wilds of the Yukon and then safely return to your home—without the people whom you would really rather not meet up with waiting on the doorstep for you? Could you vanish into the Montana ranch lands and become just another member of the local farming community? Could you melt into the masses of "street people" in New York City and not be heard of or seen again for five long years? Could you find a "doorman" willing to show you the way into the "network" of people ready to assist you in your evasion? And could you find your way onto the perfect remote Pacific island where no one cares who you are or why you came?

Those are some of the questions an evader must ask of himself if he is serious about splitting the scene for a year, 10 years, or the rest of his natural life. Ask yourself these questions. If you answered any of them with a negative or doubtful response, then take heart: by opening this book you have just taken the first step in learning how to become a successful fugitive—whether you are trying to escape from someone who is trying to kill you, or you need to break contact with your old life in order to start anew because Plan A crapped out and now your life is in turmoil (for whatever reasons).

In my primer for this book, *Fugitive: How To Run, Hide, and Survive*, I discussed the entry-level factors an evader must consider and deal with to plan and undertake a successful evasion, with emphasis on the many "little things" that can trip you up when you return to your old life. In *Advanced Fugitive* you will learn the advanced evasion techniques used successfully by evaders of all kinds to get gone and stay gone for long periods of time, perhaps forever, and we will examine in detail cases where the evaders were unsuccessful to see where they went wrong so that you won't make the same mistakes they did. Who are these evaders and what determined the outcome of their evasion? You'll learn the details of each case as you read on, but suffice it to say that military men trying to evade capture (and escaped prisoners of war struggling to remain free in enemy-held territory), accused or suspected criminals on the lam from the law, tried and convicted crooks who escaped from prison, Mafia informants running from the mob, and ordinary citizens fleeing someone trying to do them harm all contribute to the evasion wisdom you will find here.

And *Advanced Fugitive* is much more than a mere recantation of other people's evasion experiences. In the coming chapters you will learn the myriad intricacies involved in every facet of evasion, from traveling anonymously on a tramp steamer and setting in well-stocked evasion caches in any terrain (urban, suburban, or rural) to finding and using detailed instructions for changing your identity, setting snares that are difficult for searchers to detect, and exploiting the many survival assets available at no cost (and with no identification checks) to the proverbial homeless. You will also gain insight into how you can avoid having to rely on criminal elements posing as groups willing to help fugitives—which, given the deadly events of late (Waco and Ruby Ridge), the evader must elude at all costs—as well as up-to-date, practical information on some potential evasion locations outside the United States, direct from the files of the Central Intelligence Agency (CIA). There's even a complete section on the hard-core wilderness survival techniques taught to possible future evaders at the Department of Defense's (DOD's) infamous survival schools.

Let's go.

THE FUGITIVE'S WORLD
Here Be Dragons

"My ramble had sharpened my appetite, and the delicious savor of roasted meat soon rid my brains of romantic ideas."
—Osborne Russell
Journal of a Trapper

"Few things escaped his eyes. He noted the flapping flight of a raven on the horizon and the bounding fox far below."
—William O. Pruitt Jr.
Wild Harmony

This past weekend I spent some time in Washington, D.C., where I was able to tour some of America's greatest monuments, the most important of which was the Lincoln Memorial. As I stood at the massive stone feet of the great man and looked out over the reflecting pool, I was struck by how clever a survivor Lincoln was—up until one evening in the Ford Theater—and wondered how he had come by his will to persevere at all costs.

He defeated the Confederacy after a truly brutal four-year war and did so with what many military historians believe to be generals who were by and large tactically inferior to those of the South (although he did have a handful of incredibly perceptive and downright mean generals such as

William Tecumseh Sherman and Ulysses S. Grant). Lincoln had apparently decided that the North was going to win the war between the states no matter what it took, and he did just that.

When I left the Lincoln Memorial I paid my respects at The Wall (Vietnam Veterans Memorial) and then wandered past the White House on Pennsylvania Avenue. Peering through the wrought-iron fence, I could easily make out two snipers standing on the roof, both looking back at us tourists (how many of whom were actually well-armed, extremely capable Secret Service agents?) with binoculars, a sniper rifle resting on a bipod at the feet of one of the shooters. At my feet, just inside the fence, was an odd-looking device a little over a foot tall that was one of many identical devices jutting out of the lawn—listening devices, I assumed. (And where were the motion detectors and acoustic sensors hidden?) Under a tree about 30 yards away, standing in the shadow the spreading limbs made, were two additional shooters remaining very still, each dressed in black and cradling a submachine gun. (I wondered how many other like individuals were lurking on the grounds, just out of sight.) Considering all this security, I naturally wondered how far a person would get if he were to jump the fence and make a dash for the front door. Not far at all, I concluded.

Not far at all. The Secret Service is making sure that President Clinton remains a survivor.

From the White House I walked down toward the Commerce Building and watched one of Washington's seemingly innumerable homeless people eating his lunch in a bus stop shelter. He had food equivalent in calories to what most Americans eat for lunch, and he was dressed not in rags but in quite serviceable clothing. Beside him was his survival gear, strapped to one of those folding luggage haulers that you see airline flight attendants and pilots dragging their suitcases around on. His gear was completely waterproofed in apparently new heavy-duty garbage bags and was stowed carefully and securely. He probably had about 40 pounds of equipment and clothing on that rig, including a very new-looking parka. He was about five foot eight, 160 pounds or so—a decent weight for his height. His beard and long hair easily helped conceal his underlying facial features and somewhat disguised his age. The anonymous survivor.

Out on the Mall I watched another homeless man working the passersby for spare change. Of the eight people who passed him before I did, three gave him money—two dollar bills and a handful of change. That's between $2 and $3 in less than 30 seconds. Taking a low estimate of $1 per minute, that's $60 an hour, tax free. Not bad. Not bad at all. This survivor was making a living outside the system in the middle of the nation's capital, and no one cared who he was or what his story was.

All of these people—Presidents Lincoln and Clinton and the two homeless men—can be called survivors because they decided to achieve their respective goals regardless of the conditions they were or are faced with. Lincoln faced an entire army that hated him and wanted him dead, and Clinton, as do all presidents, faces the reality of a number of people who, for whatever reason, would like to kill him. But whereas two have been afforded the protection of the people, the other two have only their wits to rely upon (although, granted, those wits might lead them to soup kitchens on frequent occasions and to a homeless shelter each evening).

But the will to survive and evade detection in an urban environment does not necessarily mean one must become a quite visible street person. Indeed, one can evade in a large city with millions of inhabitants by applying evasion skills normally reserved for fugitives in wilderness areas. I know of one fugitive who built an extremely clever evasion shelter in the middle of a very large city and remained undiscovered for months on end until a single slip cost him his freedom (the smoke from his evasion fire was seen—he didn't strip the bark off the wood he was burning as he usually did; he got lazy). So the will to survive and evade capture or discovery can be applied in different ways by different people in the same place.

THE FUGITIVE'S WORLD

THE ERROR FACTOR

The hardest thing about being a fugitive is that it is so easy to make mistakes, and you can count on Murphy's Law applying to everything you say, do, and think. That is, assume that anything you say, do, or think will be held against you in the worst possible way.

Mistakes Add Up

The number and types of mistakes the fugitive can make are countless, but one of the most common is allowing your emotions to take over. For instance, in the remarkable movie *The Fugitive*, Harrison Ford plays a doctor wrongly convicted of murdering his wife. He escapes and is drawn back to the hospital in Chicago where he once worked (mistake number one—never return to your home ground if there is any way of avoiding it) and helps a young boy who was severely injured (mistake number two—although understandable, compassion can be an evasion ender). Ford is then challenged by another doctor and flees the hospital. Other mistakes he makes include trusting someone he thought was his friend who in fact was his enemy, taking an apartment when he should have lived on the street, and revealing himself to two additional hospital staffers. The fugitive was drawn back into familiar waters, and this nearly caused his demise.

In another evasion story, this one completely real, a mysterious bomber known to the authorities and the press as the "Unabomber" eluded capture for years and years while continuing his terror campaign, this despite what appears to have been the biggest, most intense manhunt in U.S. history. Finally, some seemingly insignificant mistakes and two major ones brought about his downfall.

The Federal Bureau of Investigation (FBI) alleges that Ted Kaczynski, a brilliant former professor at the University of California at Berkeley, is the Unabomber. FBI agents captured him without incident at his tiny (10-by-12-foot) ramshackle cabin near Lincoln, Montana, after being tipped off by his brother, who found some old writings of Ted's that Ted had left behind back home. The writings sounded too similar to the ravings in the Unabomber's manifesto, which had recently been published by at least two major newspapers and which Ted's brother had read.

Little mistakes Kaczynski appears to have made include keeping the typewriter he used to write the manifesto at his cabin, keeping the tools of his trade at his cabin (bomb-making materials), and patterning his movements (including a paper trail) to and from some of the bombing sites. His major mistakes were allowing his arrogance to get the best of him (the thought that he was smarter than everyone else and was therefore invincible) and writing and having published his manifesto in the first place (this was willingly handing the police a large stack of evidence).

Ted left loose ends that eventually led to his capture, and those loose ends allowed what is arguably the craftiest investigative entity in the world—the FBI—to establish an eerily accurate personality profile of Kaczynski. One break allowed the FBI to nab its alleged Unabomber, and, as with many fugitive cases, one break was all it needed. Fortunately for us, in the end, Ted's own psyche brought him down.

Don't Be Manipulated

Another easy mistake fugitives make is allowing themselves to be drawn into what appears to be a protective group of some sort. Although it is true that some groups are willing and able to provide the fugitive with assistance, there can be tremendous danger in contacting and gaining access to a group and its protection. I'm sure you recall how the folks at Waco, Jonestown, and the Freemen compound ended up.

When considering assistance from any kind of evasion group, whether it appears to be a sincere religious freedom organization in west Texas or a band of embezzling squatters on the Montana plains, the fugitive must first ask why this group exists (what is its true purpose or goal?) and secondly, why are its members willing to help (what's in it for them?).

The sad truth is, many if not most groups such as the 900-plus ill-fated residents of Jim Jones's Jonestown in Guyana,

David Koresh's assemblage of "Branch Davidian" idiots at Mt. Carmel, and the chumps who called themselves the Freemen in Montana are doomed unions. They generally consist of ill-informed and easily manipulated misfits or crooks who are nowhere near as smart as they think they are, who allow themselves to be exploited by maniacal egocentrists who are interested only in their own material, monetary, or psychological gratification (in the case of the former) or who badly underestimate their neighbors and law enforcement (in the case of the latter). The leaders of such groups are inherently dishonest and represent a dire threat to the fugitive who believes he needs their assistance.

And don't think that one of the hundreds of self-styled militias popping up around the country is your best bet. In fact, it could be your very last bet. Given events of late, such as the Oklahoma City bombing, I would be surprised if the FBI didn't have an undercover agent in every militia in America, and I know they have detailed files on them all. The last thing the fugitive needs is to show up in a group of poorly led wanna-be soldiers under the charge of a leader with questionable genuine leadership abilities who loves to hear himself rave about spectacular conspiracies and the ill-defined New World Order. Involve yourself with a group such as these, and you will find yourself compromised at the first sign of trouble. You mean less than nothing to them.

Fail to Plan and You Plan to Fail

I suspect that the most common mistake the fugitive makes is in not planning his evasion down to the last conceivable detail. An example follows.

After Pan Am flight 103 exploded over Lockerbie, Scotland, killing all aboard, a tiny fragment of the bomb allowed investigators to determine the nationality of the terrorists who planted the bomb.

Intelligence sources produced the names of two Libyan terrorists who had fled back to their lair, but, as expected, Mu'ammar al-Gadhafi refused to give them up. Now these fugitives are trapped in their own country with little hope of roaming the world again as free men. They underestimated their opponents by failing to plan their attack in a way that would allow them total and unending anonymity.

Although these two stooges were hardly world-class terrorists, even the most treacherous terrorists fail to plan for their complete protection. For instance, the Palestinian terrorist known as "The Engineer" let his guard down for just a moment, and an Israeli agent managed to get a cellular phone bomb into his hand. It disintegrated the terrorist a few seconds later.

Looking at planning from another angle, take the case of U.S. Air Force Capt. Scott O'Grady. After his F-16 was blasted from the skies over Bosnia by a Serb missile, the young officer parachuted into enemy-held territory and survived for several days by hiding "like a scared little bunny" from the hundreds of Serb killers hunting for him. Remembering his training at an air force survival school in Washington State, he moved only at night and kept to the thickest vegetation and roughest terrain he could find, slurping water from muddy puddles and eating ants as he went. He was eventually rescued by a team of specially trained Marine commandos on what is known as a TRAP (tactical recovery of aircraft and personnel) mission. O'Grady later reflected on his evasion plan of action (EPA) and how he had carefully planned for the unlikely event of his being shot down. He praised his survival instructors, too, thankful that he had paid attention during the rigorous training. This is one young man who planned to the hilt and meant to survive despite severe conditions.

TRAINING IS EVERYTHING

The fugitive must train to the point where actions become instinctive and can be undertaken after an instantaneous assessment of the situation. Reaching this level of expertise normally takes years and must encompass the full range of evasion skills: applying camouflage, finding and purifying water, navigating, building shelters, using medical techniques (including medicinal herbalism and primitive medicine), building fires, taking appropriate security measures, using clandestine communications, and defending oneself. Obviously, this is a tall order, but it is one the fugitive must work diligently to fill.

Strangely, the skill the fugitive suspects he will need the least is often the one he finds he must use to get out of a situation. This is precisely what happened to me recently.

While attending a family function with quite a few guests in attendance, I was required to deal somewhat forcefully with a large—make that *huge*—drunk who was threatening people and otherwise making a nuisance of himself. At six feet eight inches and 300 pounds, he was substantially bigger than I am and was purportedly a Vietnam vet times three and former member of the vaunted 101st Airborne, the "Screaming Eagles."

I approached the giant from the best tactical location—directly behind him—without his knowing it. (The last thing one should do in a fight is fight fair.) As he went into the attack mode, I jumped up high enough to get my left arm around his neck so that my arm could compress his external carotid artery. As I did this I turned to my right so that my left hip would jut into the small of his back as I leaned back (this increased the pressure on the artery and got him off balance). The choke hold I put on him took mere seconds to bring him down, and I remember hearing people (women) screaming ("He's killing him!") as his tongue fell out of his mouth, his eyes bulged, and his face turned a deep blue. When he became still, I released the hold and checked his carotid pulse and made sure his larynx was still in working condition (I didn't want to kill the guy, just get him under control and out of the restaurant).

Thinking about the situation the next day, I was content in the obvious realization that my training had saved me from what would no doubt have been an ugly fight—something I try to avoid—and had done so without my even thinking about it. My actions had been purely reflexive.

This is the level on which the fugitive must function, and it is a level that takes dedication to training. (At the same time, if you are in a fight then you have obviously made a serious mistake—one that could easily end your evasion.)

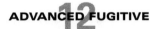

So, let's start your advanced evasion and accompanying survival training with a detailed examination of some of the world's best potential evasion areas. After all, the finest evasion and survival training in the world will be of only limited use if you fail to select the best evasion area.

WELCOME DOWN UNDERGROUND 2

"Fools say they learn from experience; I prefer to learn from the experience of others."

—Bismarck

In order to select the best possible evasion area in which you will hide and apply all the skills you will learn in this book, you must first garner a great deal of information in a wide array of areas. Let's examine some countries where you might make a go of it.

NORTH AMERICA

North America still offers quite vast tracts of land for the fugitive to take advantage of. The trick is to select the best country and region for you. Remember that a region best suited for one man may not be right for another man. Do your homework.

Canada

Canada represents one of the greatest regions on the planet for rural evasion. The country is massive and filled with many exploitable assets that the fugitive can make use of, ranging from sprawling roadless tracts of genuine wilderness complete with dense forests (35 percent of Canada is forested), in which evasion can be made substantially easier insofar as detection is concerned, to abundant water and wildlife.

Pros

By far and away, Canada's most important evasion asset for the wilderness fugitive is its sheer size coupled with wilderness regions that are difficult to access by traditional means such as vehicles. Only one region of Canada's wilderness, the Central Plains, is fairly easily accessed by truck, and because of the almost treeless nature of this stark region, the fugitive should consider other parts of Canada. (The lack of trees makes visual detection at substantial distances much more likely and the use of satellite imagery—if you are *that* hot a property—a genuine concern. Aerial photography is also more of a problem; obviously, the fugitive should not consider the Canadian Arctic icepack a viable evasion region for this same reason.)

Canada is rich in wildlife, an important consideration for the fugitive. Keep in mind that in most situations where huge herds of caribou and other highly visible animals are roaming about for all the world to see—and you might be surprised to learn how many nature buffs, photographers, scientists, tourists, and hunters find their way into areas rich in big game—the fugitive must take extra care not to be stumbled upon. Unless desperate, I would avoid the "glory" game (including, besides the aforementioned caribou, big game like elk, moose, and bears) and focus on small game like ptarmigans, ground and tree squirrels, hares, mice and voles, fish (from the smaller, less popular creeks and streams), and easily lured birds like gray jays. Small game and fish are almost always easier to take by traps and snares than big game is, and traps and snares are the preferred methods for acquiring land animals because they don't attract attention like gunfire does; fishing can be close to completely silent.

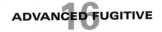

Water is another important feature of nearly all of Canada. Streams, creeks, rivers, ponds, and lakes all offer usually potable water, but do make sure you purify it regardless of the source.

With all the trees and related understory in Canada, shelter material is often readily available. A Dakota hole fire lay (see Chapter 5) using dry, barkless hardwood in a dense forest will likely go unnoticed in most areas.

The Cordillera forms Canada's western end and is divided into two sections—the Western and Eastern Cordillera. The Western Cordillera is formed by most of the Canadian Yukon, the Inuvik region, a lot of British Columbia, a section of western Alberta, and some of the Northwest Territories. The Eastern Cordillera holds 10 peaks greater than 11,500 feet in elevation, and west of the Canadian Rockies are some of the most isolated regions in Canada, including the Selkirk, Cariboo, and Stikine ranges.

Across the continent are the Maritimes—Newfoundland (and Labrador), New Brunswick, Prince Edward Island, and Nova Scotia. Of these, New Brunswick, Prince Edward Island, and much of Nova Scotia see good numbers of tourists and have the permanent population to support this tourist industry, making them largely unsuitable for the rural evader (although there are parts of Nova Scotia and New Brunswick that are certainly lightly traveled). This leaves Newfoundland. With slightly more than 405,000 square miles and a population density of only 3.6 people per square mile (the vast majority of whom are located along the coast), Newfoundland does offer the fugitive an eastern Canada option. In northern Labrador the Torngat Mountains offer good evasion possibilities.

The Canadian interior between the Rockies and the Maritimes is, like Newfoundland, populated in clusters, only in this case the clusters are major cities like Ottawa, Quebec, Sudbury, Winnipeg, Calgary, and Toronto. Quebec Province offers gigantic tracts of uninhabited forest rife with everything the fugitive would need to survive and remain hidden.

Cons

The greatest con to evading in Canada is the weather.

However, if you know how to deal with it and accept it as part of your evasion plan, the weather can even become a pro because it can thwart some people looking for you (not all, mind you, but some). The only region of Canada with weather that can in some way be considered less than extreme much of the year is coastal British Columbia, the southern part of which is a temperate rain forest. Most of the rest of Canada is subarctic and arctic. Sorry.

If you have the Royal Canadian Mounted Police looking for you, and the reason they are looking for you is because they suspect you of some crime, then you have a real problem. Forget the humorous television show about the Mountie partnered up with the American city boy—the Mounties who specialize in wilderness law enforcement are some of the most maddeningly resilient and resourceful people on the planet. If one of them makes up his mind to find you, your best bet is to leave Canada altogether. And quickly.

Most Canadians speak English as a first language (and most Quebecois speak some English), and although Canadian English is spoken with a decidedly Canadian accent, it is one Americans can easily recognize. Thus, a Canadian can just as easily recognize your American-accented English. If you run into someone in the woods who hears you speak English, he will remember you. And if he tells the Mounties and the Mounties get curious about who you are, or God forbid they suspect you of breaking their laws, well . . .

Beware of grizzly and polar bears. And falling into any of Canada's many cold waterways can make you dead from hypothermia in minutes, regardless of the season.

Vital Statistics
Land area: 9,220,970 square kilometers
Coastline: 243,791 kilometers
Climate: temperate to arctic
Currency: Canadian dollar
Languages: English and French with a smattering of native dialects

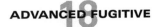

American embassy: 100 Wellington St., K1P 5T1, Ottawa/tel. (613) 238-5335/4470 (American consulates in Quebec, Toronto, Halifax, Calgary, Montreal, and Vancouver)

Rail systems: 78,148 kilometers (Surreptitiously hopping a train in remote regions can get you around very quickly; however, exercise extreme caution and remember that using trains is inherently dangerous to the fugitive.)

Mexico

Mexico represents both the very best and very worst in evasion possibilities. A large country with extremes of climate, terrain, and vegetation, Mexico has beckoned to fugitives for centuries (my paternal grandfather hunted Pancho Villa in the northern Mexican deserts), from the desert wastelands of the north to the screaming lush jungles of the south.

Pros

If I were forced to evade in Mexico and I had my choice of regions, I would select the higher mountains of the southernmost *tierra fria* (cold land). This area is substantially less arid than most of Mexico and certainly less populated than the lowlands and the coastal plains. My second choice would be the jungles of the Yucatán Peninsula, but away from the touristy areas like the Mayan pyramids.

Food and water in these regions are easy to find—there are plenty of small rodents and birds as well as small fish (though nowhere near the abundance Canada offers)—and there is vegetation available for cover in both, with the jungle clearly offering plenty of places to hide and an ecosystem that often quickly erases any sign of your passing. Triple jungle canopy protects the fugitive from satellite imagery and usually from thermal imagery as well.

Shelter in the jungle is very simple to find or create; it would be slightly more difficult to find or build an evasion shelter in the *tierra fria* because of the lack of a dense jungle to root around in. Some regions in the Yucatán are also rich in limestone caves and their related underground streams. There are no doubt countless caves in the jungle that no one knows about, and finding one is simply a matter of using a basic knowledge of geology and hydrology mixed with a little luck. Limestone caves often have narrow openings that are easily concealed, but remember that the longer you stay in one spot, the better the chances of someone detecting you or deducing your whereabouts.

Cons

With all the good things I had to say about the jungles of the Yucatán, you may be wondering why they are my second choice for evasion. The answer lies in the natural dangers of the jungle, such as snakes (the jumping pit viper is in no way amusing) and biting insects.

Mexico's desert regions are very unforgiving places, and they cover enormous amounts of territory. The fugitive evading here will soon wish he hadn't.

But aside from this, the most serious drawback to evasion south of the border is the fact that no matter where you go you are going to stick out like a sore thumb; Mexicans can spot a *gringo* a mile off, in a driving rain, on a moonless night, blindfolded. Once you have been spotted and suspicions have been aroused, you absolutely must change your location in a major way.

The language is another serious problem; as soon as you open your mouth they'll know you're an American.

Population centers like Mexico City and its massive suburbs and slums, Mérida, Chihuahua, Oaxaca, Matamoros, and Veracruz are to be avoided, as are all small towns and villages where you will definitely be remembered if seen. Street urchins, be they from remote highland villages or densely populated tourist destinations, have uncanny memories, especially when prompted with dollars. It is an unfortunate fact that most Mexicans are dirt poor, to say the least. Ten bucks will see them spill their guts—probably much less. A country full of easily bribed informants isn't an outstanding place to hide, generally speaking.

Vital Statistics
Land area: 1,923,040 square kilometers
Coastline: 9,330 kilometers
Climate: tropical to desert
Currency: new Mexican peso
Languages: Spanish (primary) with some English in tourist areas
American embassy: Paseo de la Reforma 305, Colonia Cuauhtemoc, 06500 Mexico, Distrito Federal/tel. (5) 211-0042 (consulates in Ciudad Juárez, Guadalajara, Monterrey, Tijuana, Hermosillo, Matamoros, Mérida, Nuevo Laredo)
Rail systems: 24,500 kilometers (Using the Mexican rail system illegally is extremely dangerous because of the frequency of Mexicans using it like you.)

SOUTH AMERICA

This remarkably diverse continent offers the full range of evasion possibilities, ranging from the treacherous Amazon and the towering peaks of the Andes to the extremely dangerous back streets of Lima, Peru, where packs of savage children—called "piranhas" by the locals—will audaciously descend upon you and strip you of everything of value in seconds, then leave you bleeding on the pavement. Choose wisely.

Argentina

Quite a few Nazi war criminals made it to Argentina after the war, and many hid out there successfully for many years. Argentina is an outstanding country to disappear in and is near the top of my list for many reasons.

Pros
Argentina is a large country with a history of tolerance when it comes to allowing people on the lam to take up residence there. It offers very diverse terrain, climates, and vegetation from one end to the other, and the wildlife can be prolific. The Argentines are quite sophisticated with a high literacy and

education level. They are friendly and helpful on the whole. One of the most important pros when it comes to this often visually striking country is that the population is a genuine melting pot similar to America. You could easily blend in there. Eighty-five percent of the population is white, with the remaining 15 percent being made up of Indian, mestizo, and other nonwhite groups. There are many ports for you to slip in and out of, too.

Although Spanish is the official language (which, if you don't speak it, is very easy to learn), English, German, French, and Italian are also commonly spoken. The government is more stable today than it has been in some time, and an economy that was once in major decline is rebounding well. Argentina's legal system is advanced.

The Andes form Argentina's western border with Chile and is obviously the most noted and rugged region, and if you have solid skills in alpine survival you could do well here. The *pampas* is a region of broad, fertile plains and grasslands in the northern half of the country, and survival possibilities there are good to excellent. In the south is Patagonia, which is made up of plateaus and flatlands. The fishing in Patagonia is outstanding but the weather, as in the Andes, can be tough (southernmost Patagonia is subantarctic).

Cons

As in other evasion areas, natives are going to know you are not from there as soon as you speak. This is always a drawback because they are going to remember you for a while if you interact with them in any way. The water in agricultural areas must be filtered because of the heavy use of fertilizers, herbicides, and pesticides. Flooding can be a problem in some areas (especially flash flooding below the mountains), and sudden, fierce windstorms called *pamperos* are a threat on the *pampas*. The southwest is arid and the southeast is subantarctic.

Vital Statistics
Land area: 2,736,690 square kilometers

Coastline: 4,989 kilometers
Climate: temperate with highly regionalized extremes of desert and subantarctic
Currency: nuevo peso Argentino
Languages: Spanish (official), with English being commonly spoken
American embassy: 4300 Colombia, 1425 Buenas Aires/tel. (1) 777-4533/4534
Rail systems: with 34,572 kilometers of rail, trains are a pretty good option for getting around

I don't recommend any other countries in South America because of stability problems, loose lips that start to flap for a few dollars, and health risks caused by disease.

THE EASTERN ATLANTIC, EUROPE, AND SCANDINAVIA

Perhaps the best thing about this piece of the planet is the fact that, insofar as general appearance is concerned, a caucasion can blend in well, with little effort. But as is the case just about everywhere else, your language abilities are what will trip you up the easiest, not what you look like.

The British Isles

England, Ireland, and Scotland are always a solid choice for evasion, but forget finding vast tracts of wilderness; they are long gone. Nevertheless, you could start a new life in an out-of-the-way town or small city and just fade into the background. Avoid trying to blend into the populace in small villages where everyone knows everyone else and the pubs are filled with talkative, gregarious people who love to speculate on the Yank living on the McKenzie farm. Remember John Wayne in *The Quiet Man*? You saw how fast the word got around that an American was about, right?

London, Manchester, Birmingham, Glasgow, and Dublin are all potential evasion cities. Avoid Belfast and the rest of Northern Ireland, for obvious reasons.

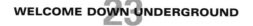

If you decide on Wales, Scotland, or Ireland, select a new name that matches the population, and come up with a cover story that reflects your ancestry from that region. The Irish especially are very prone to taking in and accepting long-lost sons of Ireland who have returned "home" after perhaps centuries of their end of the family's being in America or Canada (saying you are Canadian instead of American is often a good ploy because it further muddies the water where your tracks lie on the bottom). The Welsh, Irish, and Scots all have ironclad memories and pride themselves on this fact; change your appearance in a big way to throw anyone looking for you off your trail.

Although you could disappear into the London counterculture somewhat easily and never be found, let's focus on Ireland.

Pros

Ireland has the ability to swallow up someone who endears himself to a community, especially if, as previously stated, you make yourself out to be a long-lost son of the emerald isle returning home, never to leave again. The temperate maritime climate makes for winters that are quite mild (although it can at times get cold) and cool summers. Gray skies are the norm about one out of every two days.

The Irish terrain in the interior is flat or gently rolling; on the west coast there are striking sea cliffs, and on the east coast there are low mountains and hills.

With Ireland's very stable government and strong work ethic (although unemployment remains a major problem at 16 percent), the fugitive who finds his way to Ireland could get by in some out-of-the-way town as a laborer of some sort, or perhaps on a commercial fishing boat. Better yet, develop your photography skills and become self-employed. (Having a skill that you can bring with you that allows you to be self-employed is an outstanding asset for the fugitive.) If you scored a fairly generous chunk of money somehow, you could buy a cottage somewhere in the middle of nowhere special and hunker down for a spell. If you are any shade of white you will likely be able to blend right in with the populace, and if you have blue or green eyes and hair with a reddish tinge, you're looking good. (Don't forget that designer contacts and hair coloring can work wonders.)

Cons

For evasion in the wilderness, Ireland leaves a lot to be desired because the island is 71 percent pasture, meadow, and field; only 5 percent of Ireland is forested to any degree. Also, heavy chemical use on agricultural land has created a problem with water purity in all the streams and lakes accepting runoff. Purify all water taken from these sources.

Ireland has a huge tourist trade, and it is conceivable that bad luck might get you recognized by someone on vacation. Your accent is going to give you away immediately, so work on it.

Vital Statistics

Land area: 70,280 square kilometers
Coastline: 1,448 kilometers
Climate: temperate maritime
Currency: Irish pound
Languages: English (official), Gaelic
American embassy: 42 Elgin Road, Ballsbridge, Dublin/tel. (1) 668-7122
Rail systems: with the country's nearly 2,000 miles of rail, the fugitive can get around well

Germany

Germany grew substantially landwise when East and West became one in October of 1990. They've had some growing pains, but the German people are extremely unlikely to allow any long-term problems associated with the merging to bring them down.

Centrally located in Europe, Germany is a diverse nation (lots of Turks and Americans) with nationalistic tendencies that will never go away. I have spent a great deal of time there and know the country and its people well, and even though Germans like Germans best, they do accept others if you go out of your way to get into and respect the German way of life. Because of Germany's location in Europe it is easy to travel from there to other countries, especially via rail. Germany shares borders with Austria, Belgium, the Czech Republic, Denmark, France, Luxembourg, Netherlands, Poland, and Switzerland. A good way to disappear in Germany is to have your name officially changed and cover your tracks as you do so (Paladin Press's catalog offers a wide selection of books on how to do this), then get a fresh American passport and go there (skip the false passport because the German *polizie* are likely to immediately recognize it as a phony).

Pros

The biggest pro when it comes to evasion in Germany is one's ability to move around easily within the country and from there into the rest of Europe without records being kept of who went where when. The best places to evade in Germany are the major cities, where you can melt into the populace; small towns have people who like to talk at the local *gasthaus*, which is a bar.

Work is readily available in Germany, but being self-employed is the way to go. A job that doesn't keep you in one place and allows you to make do financially without having to report income to a government agency is preferable.

English is widely spoken, but for faster cooperation, speak German first when greeting someone. The Germans like it when you try and will respect you for it, even if you butcher it pretty badly.

Germany has a large tourist industry, so it is easy for you to just be another unremarkable tourist on holiday.

Cons

Forget wilderness evasion. Although the Alps might appear perfect for evasion to the uninitiated, the German people traipse over every square inch of them on a regular basis, and woodsmen, farmers, and hunters know the land very well; they'll likely know it if you are nearby or have recently passed through their woods or fields.

Germany has problems with air pollution that forms acid

rain and river pollution from industrial waste, so all water must be purified.

Some foreigners have had problems with gangs of neo-Nazi youths who want to rid Germany of all people who aren't German. They have attacked and in some cases killed foreigners. Be wary.

Vital Statistics
Land area: 356,910 square kilometers
Coastline: 2,389 kilometers
Climate: temperate and maritime—summers are cool and wet, and winters are cooler and wet, with much snowfall in the Alps
Currency: Deutsche mark
Languages: German (official). English is widely spoken to some degree. French and Italian are also spoken near those borders.
American embassy: Deichmanns Aue 29, 53170 Bonn/tel. (228) 2663. Consulate(s) General in Frankfurt, Hamburg, Leipzig, Munich, and Stuttgart.
Rail systems: 43,457 kilometers and highly reliable

Norway

If you are entertaining ideas of wilderness evasion in a cold foreign land, Norway is for you. With large expanses of nearly unpopulated terrain, this home of the Vikings is rich in possibilities.

Pros

An expert in subarctic or arctic alpine survival would find northern Norway much to his liking. The southwestern coast, on the other hand, is less extreme. Glaciers abound in the north, and the interior is very mountainous with fjords along the coast. Tundra is found in the far north. Yes, all of these things, to the expert, are pros.

Wildlife is quite abundant to prolific in some areas. Fish are plentiful. About 27 percent of the country is forested, and when you add those forests to the rugged mountains you get an area that can easily intimidate someone coming after you.

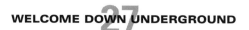

Cons

If you aren't up to the task, surviving the climate and terrain can be a killer. English is not widely spoken, even in Oslo. Water pollution from acid rain is a growing problem. Norway has many towns and villages, usually situated on the coast or a river, and people tend to notice and remember strangers.

Vital Statistics

Land area: 324,220 square kilometers
Coastline: 21,925 kilometers
Climate: Temperate along both coasts (although the west coast sees more precipitation), colder in the interior, and tundra in the far north, where the Lapps live and herd reindeer
Currency: Norwegian krone
Languages: Norwegian (official). Lapp and Finnish in isolated pockets.
American embassy: Drammensveien 18, 0244 Oslo/tel. 22 44 85 50
Rail systems: 4,026 kilometers (and you can easily jump a train in remote areas to get around)

There are innumerable other places to evade to in the world, with interesting opportunities on the many islands in the western Pacific of particular note. The Caribbean also offers some island possibilities, especially those that are more popular with Europeans than Americans. Eastern Europe, Asia, and the Orient don't have much to offer, realistically speaking. You can easily conduct research on the Internet/World Wide Web by simply going to a search engine (Yahoo!, Excite, Magellan, and so on) and typing in the name of the country you want to learn about. Or just head for the library, but don't check any books out; you could easily be traced if you do so. Read the book there and split.

DEATH FROM AFAR
Avoiding and Countering the Sniper

> "A knowledge of the elementary principles of movement and concealment in hostile territory is essential."
> —Lt. Col. Rex Applegate
> *Kill or Get Killed*

The feeling of being pursued is intense, to say the least. Anyone who has ever played football and been chased by one or more opponents while running the ball knows the feeling and how adrenaline kicks in to make the legs pump at a remarkable rate. Now imagine what it would be like to be pursued by someone who wants to not only *catch* you, but *keep* you caught for his own purposes. Moreover, imagine being *hunted* by a man with a high-powered rifle equipped with a telescopic sight who wants not to capture you but *kill* you. And this man is extremely well trained, possessing an almost psychotic sense of mission accomplishment.

This man may be the fugitive's worst nightmare—the professional sniper.

WHO AND WHAT YOU'RE UP AGAINST

What causes an ordinary man to become an extraordinary sniper—a fine-tuned killing machine who knows no quarter and expects none; a man who will go to any length, to any extreme, to kill his target with one shot to the head or heart fired at several hundred, sometimes thousands of yards? What makes a man want to blow someone's head off from a great distance, sometimes only for the satisfaction that he was able to do so and get away with it unscathed and undetected?

The answers lie deep within the sniper's psyche, where dwells man's most primitive emotions, desires, and needs. Herein lies the desire to survive, to continue living. And it is this desire that turns a normal human being into a man who sometimes plays important roles in the shaping of events both local and global, personal and public. Linked to this desire is, from time to time, the emotion called hatred. Oftentimes it is this emotion that causes the sniper to cross the line from being a legitimate law enforcement or military sharpshooter such as

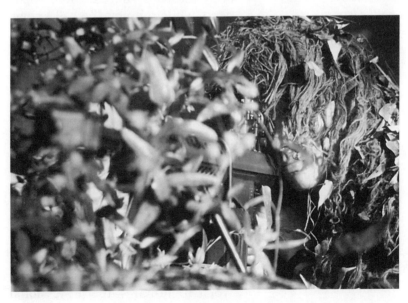

The sniper has long played critical roles in countless contests.

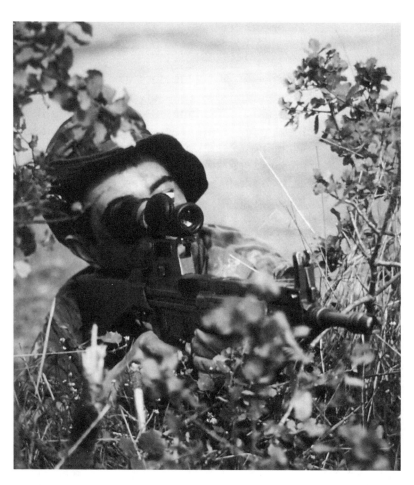

One shot is all he needs.

Gunnery Sergeant Carlos Hathcock II (Ret.) to a twisted killer such as Lee Harvey Oswald. But no matter what the sniper's mind-set, if he is after you and he is a professional meaning to kill you at all costs, you, the fugitive, are in genuine mortal danger. The steps you take to avoid being tracked, spotted, stalked, or fired upon by the sniper—and those you take to counter his fire—will determine the outcome of your evasion. There is absolutely no margin for error when you are trying to thwart the actions or counter the fire of the sniper. One mistake and you become a number for the sniper to add to his list of confirmed kills.

The most effective snipers—the ones who seldom if ever miss while racking up impressive numbers and making incredible shots under the most demanding of conditions—are those who operate in two-man teams. The world's most proficient snipers, those belonging to the U.S. Marines, have operated in two-man teams for decades and have amassed astonishing success records in wars around the globe. Carlos Hathcock, widely accepted as the most dangerous sniper ever created, usually operated as half of a two-man team and amassed 93 confirmed kills and hundreds of probables while serving as a sniper in Vietnam. The reason snipers operate in two-man teams is simple: two pairs of highly trained eyes are twice as efficient as one pair.

As the fugitive, then, you are going to be required to avoid two snipers who function as one implacable entity. Yes, both members of the sniper team are fully trained in all aspects of their craft—double jeopardy for the fugitive.

Training

The modern law enforcement or military sniper is formally (school) trained and has had extensive on-the-job training and experience. The criminal sniper employed by organized crime is likely to have had military marksmanship training and possibly formal sniper training as well, or he may even be a former law enforcement officer gone astray. No matter what organization the sniper belongs to at the moment, you can rest assured that he is a devoted professional who abhors defeat, errors, and tactical mistakes. Any sniper is able to engage a fugitive accurately at ranges up to and sometimes slightly exceeding 1,000 yards. And with upgraded weapons systems like the Barrett M82A1 Special Application Scoped Rifle (SASR, a .50-caliber sniper rifle), he can reach out and touch someone at distances in the 2,000-yard range and then some. (I personally witnessed graphically accurate shots on unsuspecting Iraqis with this weapon at 1,800+ yards in the Gulf War—not a pretty sight, although I will say that such sights are certainly memorable.)

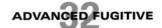

Besides being able to shoot the eyes out of a rattlesnake at a thousand yards and not bruise the lids, modern snipers are masters of total camouflage under any conditions—urban, suburban, and rural. They can splatter you from the natural concave shadow of a hotel room as you walk down the street a grid square away just as easily as they can dump you from a belly or stump hide overlooking a forest clearing.

Personal Attributes

The personal attributes of professional snipers include the following:

- intelligent
- crafty
- decisive
- aggressive
- calm under extreme stress
- mentally stable
- highly capable with a map and compass, as well as being proficient in primitive navigation and survival techniques
- in excellent physical condition (possessing impressive stamina)
- highly disciplined
- very self-confident
- mature
- independent thinking

Dealing with a polished marksman who possesses all these attributes and is hunting you is obviously going to take extreme prejudice and cunning.

Support Equipment

The sniper's support equipment is likely to consist of the following:

- night vision/sighting devices
- a secondary rifle such as an M16A2 (carried by the spotter, i.e., the second man in the team)

- sidearms (normally semiautomatic pistols)
- powerful binoculars
- a spotting scope
- fighting knives
- communications equipment

Camouflage

The camouflage a sniper chooses to make himself appear as just another part of the terrain runs the gamut from extremely simple to remarkably clever. It takes into account the following eight factors of complete camouflage:

- shine
- shadow
- movement
- color
- contrast
- texture
- shape
- tone

His camouflage may consist of a ghillie suit (a loose-fitting smock that covers the sniper from head to foot, made of assorted pieces of cloth designed to completely disrupt his shape and blend in perfectly with the surrounding vegetation) or some other complex outfit, or it may simply be a set of camouflage utilities with a little natural vegetation added. Whatever it is, the professional sniper will be sure to apply every principle of camouflage to his movements and positions.

THE SNIPER'S DEEP BAG OF TRICKS

The lengths to which the sniper will go to get you are phenomenal. But while the sniper's bag of treacherous tricks may be seemingly bottomless, the fugitive can get the upper hand on him by anticipating his arrival and actions and then deceiving or tricking him in such a way that he becomes exposed long enough to be dispatched by the fugitive, falls prey to a fatal booby trap, or decides that the fugitive is not in that area. The key to all this is to be thinking like the sniper *before* he shows up in your area and kill him *before* he ever gets wind or sight of you. If he gets you in the crosshairs first, it's end game.

Time-Honored Observation Techniques

One of the sniper's greatest assets is his (or his team's) ability to detect engageable targets. The two primary senses he uses to locate a target are sight and sound, and, to a lesser degree, he uses smell.

Sight

Most targets are located because of their failure to be totally camouflaged, meaning that they have failed to apply all eight camouflage factors to completely hide themselves. All the sniper needs is one tiny mistake, and he will likely make the kill. Carlos Hathcock, in one of his most memorable engagements, made a kill on North Vietnam's top sniper, who just so happened to be hunting Carlos (the gunny was not very popular with the North Vietnamese Army or Vietcong and had a bounty placed on his head by the enemy, which the enemy sniper was trying hard to collect). Carlos and his spotter knew they were being hunted, and the enemy sniper knew they were hunting him. As the opponents slithered into shooting position and began searching for a target, Carlos' rifle swung onto something that didn't look quite natural. Peering through the scope, he detected something round in the center of his crosshairs—he was looking straight into the scope of the enemy sniper, who was looking straight into Carlos's scope. Hathcock instantly squeezed the trigger.

The bullet flew right down the enemy sniper's scope and into his head, exiting in the back and killing the man on the spot. Carlos and his spotter (who was later killed in action) carefully approached the place where they believed the sniper had been and found the man's body, minus a large portion of the back of his head. Hathcock has since reflected that the only reason he was alive was because he "got on the trigger first."

But the enemy sniper would never have been killed as he

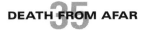

was if he had been completely camouflaged, even though there was only one miniscule portion of his camouflage that was left unattended to. Carlos's keen eyes picked up the mistake and ended the contest.

Improper movement is oftentimes the mistake a target makes. Movement draws the human eye like a magnet. The fugitive, when moving, must make all his movements slowly and deliberately. The faster he moves, the better the chances of his being detected. (Crawling and other movement techniques will be discussed later in this book.) Besides improper movement, contrast, shine, and the fugitive's outline are three of the most common giveaways.

Sound

There are many natural sounds in the wild, but the sniper keys in on those sounds that are suspicious or obviously human, the most obvious of which is the human voice. The fugitive must learn to use the natural sounds of his evasion areas to mask the sounds he makes. Windy days when brush and other vegetation are moving and creating noise are often prime movement days—*if* you must move during daylight hours (night is absolutely the best time to move about, especially when it's raining). Using the sound of a running stream or river to mask your sounds is also wise.

Gear and clothing must be made as soundproof as possible prior to any movement, regardless of the external conditions.

Smell

The human olfactory isn't the sharpest sense, but it is capable of detecting some surprisingly subtle smells. Food, smoke, urine, and feces are familiar odors to our noses, and the sniper uses his sense of smell to detect sign the fugitive left or even the fugitive himself.

Food should be cooked quickly and eaten immediately to reduce smell. Smoke from fires can be greatly reduced by using the Dakota hole (see Chapter 5) with properly prepared fuel. Body waste disposal is covered later in this chapter.

Deception

The art of deception is a game of making the fugitive come to a false conclusion. The fugitive must be extremely conscious and suspicious of tricks. For instance, one of the oldest tricks in the book, used to lure a target into a kill zone being watched by the sniper, is to have a couple of apparently harmless passers-by make their presence known to the fugitive by talking, sitting around a campfire, or what have you. They stay in a spot or small area long enough (and make just enough noise) to get the fugitive's attention, who naturally just spies on them. Eventually they leave but are sure to leave behind—apparently accidentally—something in the open and clearly visible that the fugitive is likely to want, such as some food or equipment. The fugitive waits until he feels sure the party has left the area and sneaks down to the object. He is then shot by the sniper.

Never take anything left in your evasion area by anyone, no matter how long ago it was left there. A good sniper will continually check on something left behind to see if it has disappeared. If a set of binos or a can of Spam suddenly vanishes after sitting on a log for three weeks, he'll know you are in the area and will likely be able to track you from there. At this point it is probably only a matter of time before he kills you.

Modern Technological Tools

Modern technology is the bane of the fugitive. Nowadays there are several reliable sources that anyone can tap to acquire devices designed to detect people trying to hide.

Seismic Sensors

Seismic sensors are devices, always camouflaged to appear like bushes, shrubs, or other natural vegetation, that use geophones implanted in the ground that detect vibrations made by things moving near them. These very sensitive sensors can easily detect a man walking or crawling by who isn't using the utmost in stealth movement techniques.

Ground Surveillance Radar (GSR)

Ground surveillance radar (radio detecting and ranging)

detects movement of people or objects that are in the line of sight of the device. This means that anyone or anything moving within the radar's range and not masked by a terrain feature or heavy vegetation of some sort can be detected.

The fugitive can thwart GSR by moving very slowly and very low to the ground. This plays on the technical abilities of the radar operator who, unless extremely experienced and remarkably gifted in the operation of the set, will be unable to recognize the fugitive's movements. This radar is also unable to detect anyone or anything outside of its direct line of sight. So if the fugitive remains in defilade—using terrain features like ridges, eskers, knolls, and hills—the radar will be useless.

Night Vision Devices (Passive and Active)

Night vision devices (NVDs) have improved by leaps and bounds over the last 20 years. Many of today's NVDs are extremely reliable and efficient. There are two types: passive, which amplify existing light from any source (the stars and moon, streetlights, headlights), and active, which use artificial light created by the device itself.

Passive devices such as the old "starlight" scope have their uses but are limited because of weather conditions (cloud cover, rain). Active devices are more reliable because the weather does not affect their capabilities.

The fugitive who uses stealthy movement techniques and anticipates the operators of the NVDs can foil them. He must stay in dense vegetation and move very slowly. He must never stand up, crawling everywhere he suspects NVDs are in use. He must avoid natural avenues of approach like paths, game trails, roads, and clearings, which are likely to be monitored. Perfect camouflage and movement techniques will keep the fugitive hidden.

Infrared Heat Detection Devices (IHDDs)

This equipment is one of the most serious threats to the fugitive. IHDDs use thermal imaging to detect anyone and anything giving off heat exceeding that of the surrounding environment. Perfect standard visual camouflage and total stillness are not enough to beat these systems.

In my evasion classes, I teach potential fugitives to use heat reflection material such as backpacker's space blankets, which are available in any good camping store. Constructed of Mylar or some similar material like paper-thin (and specially treated) aluminum and quite light, the space blanket reflects the body's heat back toward it rather than allowing it to escape and be "seen" by an IHDD. In the Hollywood version of this, Arnold Schwarzeneggar coats himself with mud in *Predator* to render the integrated IHDD belonging to that "ugly mudda fucka" useless. The principle behind this act is valid.

Tracking Skills

Professional snipers are master trackers in all situations. Their powers of observation and deduction are outstanding. This means that the fugitive is going to have to become incredibly clever when it comes to not leaving any sign for the sniper/tracker to cut, i.e., he must leave no sign of his passing.

I have been taught by some astonishingly gifted trackers and can attest to their uncanny ability to deduce accurately almost unbelievable amounts of information from a single print or other clue. A good tracker can deduce your height, weight, general age, physical condition, type and weight of gear, time of passage, speed of travel, mind-set (scared, calm, nervous), nationality, estimated current position, and level of survival and evasion training. Impossible, you say? How could it be possible to tell a man's height? If you have ever walked through the woods in spring, summer, or early fall, you have accidentally walked through spider webs stretched between trees. An observant tracker looks for such sign. Sure, a bat or bird or moose might have gone through the web, but the tracker checks for corroborating sign at the site.

Insofar as leaving no sign goes, individual prints (or parts thereof), sets of prints, damaged vegetation, and manmade items are frequently the most common evidence of your having been there. By avoiding walking or otherwise moving over soft earth or mud and sticking to hard earth and perhaps certain types of leaf litter—although the latter won't fool the best trackers—the fugitive can minimize but never truly eliminate sign.

The tracker often finds manmade items like bits of food (or its containers), cigarette butts (quit smoking; it's too much of a liability), chewing gum, old batteries, and so on, and these frequently act as starting points for the final phases of the tracker's mission. Brush moved aside must be returned to its original position, and no leaves, twigs, shoots, or other parts of a plant can be harmed (and this includes leaving no rubs on the stalk where your fingers might have grasped it or where the edge of your hand might have pushed it aside). When climbing a steep bank, don't use vegetation to pull yourself up—the pressure will damage the plant, and the loosed stalk base, bent shaft, grip marks, or rubs will be detectable to the well-trained eye.

When getting water, never expose yourself on the bank and never attempt it during the day. Instead, fasten your cup or canteen or water bottle to a pole and carefully push it out from the brush into the water, at night. If you are foraging for plants—an extreme likelihood when evading in the wild—never leave any part of a foraged plant anywhere to be seen. If the plant is small enough, take the whole thing, fill in the hole so that it looks natural (like there was never a plant there in the first place), and hide the parts you don't eat under a log or rock (but leave no sign at the hiding place). If you are foraging parts off a large tree that can't be moved, such as some terminal growth from a cedar or pine, make it look like an animal did it. For example, I keep the skeletal jaw of a whitetail deer in my evasion kit. If I need to forage a plant that deer eat, I find one of those plants where they have been feeding and use the jaw to snip off the terminal growth so that it looks like just another deer nibble, and I'm sure to leave no footprints. I also have a hare jaw for low-to-the-ground plants. When using this tactic it is important to remember to take parts of plants that the animal you are imitating does in fact eat; a crafty tracker will recognize the ruse if you foul up.

Campfires tell a great deal. The fugitive must never build a fire that can be seen by anyone but himself. Again, see Chapter 5 for details.

Any animal or fish carcasses you end up with must be dis-

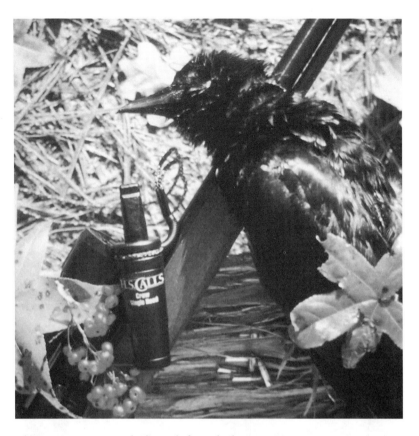

This crow's carcass must be disposed of completely.

posed of with great caution. If you just toss them into streams, they can float downstream and be found by the tracker, who now knows that you are upstream. Here's another reason to catch only small land animals and fish if they are plentiful enough to sustain you: the carcass of a squirrel is much easier to get rid of than that of a caribou, and the carcass of a brook trout is much easier to rid yourself of than that of a 30-pound catfish. But still, a body of water is often the best place to dispose of a carcass. Trying to hide carcass parts on land can go bad when a critter smelling the parts discovers them, digs them up (assuming you buried them in some way), and leaves them

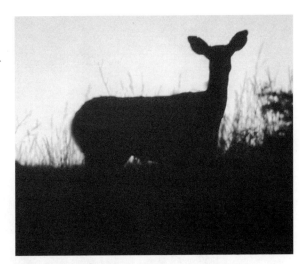

Right: The carcass of a deer is more difficult to hide than that of small game.

Below: Small fish carcasses, on the other hand, are easy to get rid of.

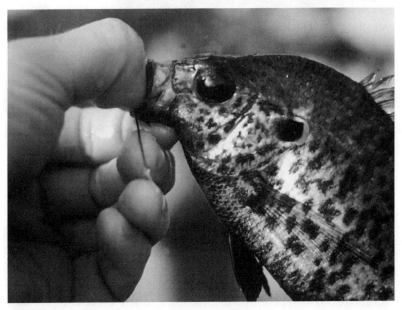

exposed for the tracker to find and decipher. The water should be as deep as possible, and the carcass should be securely weighted with a rock and sunk in the water away from the bank. Running water will help mask the splash of the rock when you toss it, as can the presence of wind or rain. Use a rock that is just big enough to further reduce splash.

When cleaning a critter, the fugitive must use the greatest caution to avoid leaving blood, bones, and other body parts at the cleaning site. Again, water is your best bet. (Place a rock taken from the water—don't leave a visible hole in the streambed or riverbed—on top of the guts and carcass; creatures in the water will eat it quickly in most cases.) By cleaning all fish and game on a moonless night along a heavily vegetated bank, you can solve the problem of being easily spotted.

Then there is the problem of dealing with human waste. This is one of the fugitive's easiest things to gaff off, and it can be his last. Urine must be deposited in a small hole at least eight inches deep and then covered over so that it appears nothing ever happened there, or it can go into a stream or creek. Feces must always go into a hole at least a foot deep and then be covered in the same manner. An option is to move a small log aside gingerly, scrape out a hole in the depression the log made (making sure none of the dirt and detritus leaves the depression), doing your business in the hole, filling the hole back in, and then replacing the log. You must be sure the log did not leave any sign of its having been moved. And while this may or may not have you cringing a little, it needs to be said: defecating in the water is to be avoided, since the feces may float.

THE COUNTERSNIPER

This is you.

The best countersnipers are snipers themselves. They think and act just like the guy gunning for them. This means that they have all the knowledge and abilities their opponent has. They are expert shots under all conditions, can detect targets regardless of the situation, and have a solid grasp of shooting positions, camouflage, range estimation, weather effects on bullet flight, trigger control, observation, movement, tracking, and stalking. Also, they have a very accurate rifle and the right ammunition to go with that rifle—namely, match ammo or special hand loads.

What all this means to the fugitive is that besides being able to hide, he must be able to hunt someone who is hunting him and kill that someone with a single shot at ranges up to 1,000 yards. Clearly this requires some serious training in sniping skills, and such training is available. (See Appendix A for a list of schools.)

Let's move on.

LIFE ON THE STREET
The Concrete Jungle

4

"He who would win should not suffer from moral inhibitions."
—Gen. Waldemar Erfurth
Surprise

In the 1940s and 1950s, street people or "the homeless" were referred to as derelicts, bums, vagrants, and, if they got around by hitching unauthorized rides on freight trains, hobos. Then, with the advent of the hippie era in the late 1960s, people who hung out on the street in such quaint locales as Haight-Ashbury in the city by the bay, San Francisco—many of whom are apparently still there along with their progeny, who have no clue what it was really like to grow up in the sixties but who try hard to pretend they do—became looked upon as poor, wretched, lost, and misguided individuals who just couldn't grasp the 20th century with any fervor to speak of. Nowadays they are called *homeless*, and they are found in every state from coast to coast, living however they can on whatever they can.

What a bunch of crap.

The truth of the matter is that these losers almost always live at the expense of taxpayers like you and me. Most have decent clothing, eat at least two meals a day (I generally eat one meal a day), sleep without rain and snow pelting them, and have a reliable source of income, that being, of course, you and me, either through taxes or responsible adult-to-scumbag handouts, i.e., giving beggars money.

Every society since the Roman empire has had its losers, and we are no different today. The good part about all this is that you, the fugitive, can play directly off our liberal society by becoming just another faceless, nameless, well-fed, warm, and dry *homeless* person for as long as you need to remain in that status. If you play your role correctly, no one will bother you, interrogate you, suspect you, question you, wonder about you, or concern themselves in any way with you except for feeding you, housing you, clothing you, and arranging for your medical and dental needs.

What a deal!

BLENDING INTO THE BACKGROUND

If your evasion plan of action calls for you to become one of the homeless, so to speak, you are going to have to blend into the background, i.e., look and act no different than any of the genuine losers beside you on the street (or park bench, as the case may be). This means that you are probably going to have to alter your appearance, actions, and demeanor somewhat.

Appearance

Your appearance is going to have to be changed as radically as possible from what you used to look like back before your life got turned upside down. If you had no facial hair in your old life, now you must grow some, preferably plenty of it. What was once short hair must become longish, and vice versa. If you used to wear glasses but not contact lenses, change to contact lenses (and consider getting a pair in a color other than your true eye color). If you didn't wear eyeglasses, pick up a couple of pairs of plain glass (no prescription) glasses with not-too-flashy rims—just plain old glasses.

Got any tattoos? Get rid of them by visiting a surgeon who specializes in their removal, but do so away from your current place of residence and pay cash for the service (use false identification, too). Scars, too, can lead to your being identified, so do whatever you can to hide or alter them.

Consider the use of other props, like an old cane or walking stick that helps your newfound limp. A slight danger exists here in that someone seeing a man hobbling along with a cane or walking stick is likely to remember that person more than a guy who wasn't crippled.

You must abandon all your old clothing. "New" old clothing can be picked up cheap from charitable organizations and at yard and garage sales, but always shop for these items out of town. Buy drab, unremarkable clothing, pay in cash, and wear and say nothing that would make someone remember you. Park your car well away from where you do your actual shopping to minimize the chances of someone seeing and remembering what you drove.

Do you speak with an accent? Practice speaking without it (this can take less time than you might think if you really set your mind to it and practice). The same can be said for picking up an accent. My repertoire of accents include southern, upper midwest (with a hint of German), down east (Maine), southern Californian (Dude! Like, this is a major bummer, man, cuz, like, the mall is closed!), eastern European, French Canadian, Long Island yuppie, west Texas redneck, born-and-raised haoli Hawaiian, southie Boston, Cedar Island (the dialect spoken by watermen indigenous to the Cedar Island region of Carteret County, North Carolina, who are from mostly Scottish stock), and several others. But here are two warnings: first, practice enough to become very comfortable with the accent (enough so to be able to stick to it under duress, i.e., an interrogation) and, second, acquire a Social

Security number from the region you are imitating the accent of. Social Security cards are issued by region! For instance, someone from central Florida who applies for a Social Security number there will get a number starting with 265 or thereabouts. If you are speaking with a Boston accent while answering police officers' questions, but your Social Security number says you got it while living in Nebraska, you are going to have to explain the inconsistency. I have found that the less conversation you have in an interrogation, the better.

Actions and Demeanor

How you act while "homeless" is just as critical to your subterfuge as your appearance and language/accent. The trick is to act like most of the other homeless people while avoiding acting in any way that will draw attention to yourself or cause passersby or anyone you are interacting with to remember things about you that someone looking for you can use. The key is to be subtle. The late William Colby, former head of the CIA and a genuine spy himself in his early days with the OSS, once remarked that his appearance was that of the perfect spy: he could walk into a room full of people and no one would notice him or remember his having been there once he had left. This ability is your goal. However, it can be easier said than done depending on your outward appearance, personality, and life experiences. For instance, I can easily adjust my personality to become no one special, but my features make it easy for people to remember me (my weathered appearance tells intuitive people that I have spent much time exposed to the elements). Also, because of my life experiences, I continuously check others out, observe their actions, and generally remain extremely aware of what is going on around me—which, again, tends to make observant people notice me. These are attributes that are at the same time detractors to the fugitive in certain circumstances.

Generally speaking, the perspicacious fugitive acting as just another hapless homeless person is the way to go. I recommend avoiding playing the mentally ill, babbling, mumbling homeless weirdo. When it comes time to ask for money

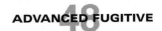

from kindhearted passersby, it is more productive to smile and ask directly for some change or a dollar for "an old veteran" or "an American temporarily down on his luck" and then thank them as they continue by than it is to just act like the village idiot while hunched over like some freak out of *The Hunchback of Notre Dame*, shaking a cup of change at people and grunting.

The art of begging shows that the latter is often perceived as a potential threat by people walking by and will be avoided, while more friendly beggars take in all the cash. When someone walking a few steps behind another sees you thank that person for giving you a dollar, he is more likely to chip in as well because you are not a threat and are courteous. Americans love harmless, courteous people and shy away from strange, rude people.

SELECTING YOUR NEW HOMETOWN: THINGS TO CONSIDER

Your new hometown should offer as many amenities as possible and be removed from any other places you have ever lived, including places where you grew up; it is just too easy to be recognized by people you haven't seen in decades in a town or city you haven't been in for just as long. Never trust your luck.

A careful reconnaissance of the city whose streets you are considering inhabiting is called for. The last thing you need as a street person is to try to survive and evade in a city that is inhospitable to you and your kind.

Weather

There is probably no need for you to hit the streets of a northern city known for severe winters, such as Minneapolis/St. Paul, Fargo, Boston, Buffalo, Duluth, Detroit, or Chicago. Why put up with freezing cold and brutal blizzards when you might be able to just as easily move to warmer climes, in cities such as Miami, Orlando, Atlanta, Birmingham, Dallas, Houston, Phoenix, Albuquerque, Los Angeles, San Diego, El Paso, and Ft. Lauderdale? Just because you are on the street doesn't mean you must also be miser-

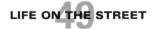

able. Misery of any physical kind isn't a requirement in leading the life of a homeless person.

Societal Attitudes

Some cities take a very tolerant attitude toward the homeless, while others are openly hostile toward them. To find out what the attitude is in a potential evasion city, call the mayor's office and explain to the appropriate person that you are a wealthy businessman considering moving your firm to that city and that you would like to know what the city's policies are toward the homeless, i.e., does the city coddle them or does the city take measures to keep them at arm's length? Then call the local chapter of the American Civil Liberties Union (ACLU) and ask them for their opinion. You want the city that coddles the homeless; the last thing you need is to be rousted by the fuzz.

Check out all the agencies and organizations in place to assist the homeless. The mayor's office can give you a list of shelters, churches, and missions that help the homeless, as well as a list of so-called soup kitchens and free medical clinics. The more the merrier. Cities with few such amenities are likely to have comparatively few homeless (or an *attitude* towards them), which will make you more vulnerable to recognition by not having enough "background" to blend into.

Race Relations

Check into the demographics of the city; the homeless population will likely reflect the demographics of the population at large. If you are white and the overwhelming majority of homeless in a certain city is not, there may be a racial problem there—one that would put you at a disadvantage.

GEARING UP

Street survival clothing and equipment in many ways parallel the gear you would need for surviving in the wild, but your gear has to lend itself well to staying on the move; the fugitive must never sleep in the same place two nights in a row. In fact, a good general rule for sleeping locations is to never use the same location more than once in a 30-day period. This way you avoid patterning yourself too tightly.

Clothing

Your clothing—everything from your socks and underwear to your coats and hat—should appear well-used but serviceable—not ratty, but not brand new either. (Remember, one of the things that drew my attention to the Washington bum in the bus stop shelter was his new-looking parka.) No clothing should have any type of logo or wording on it, since these things make items of clothing easier to remember. Drab colors like gray, brown, beige, dark blue, and black are preferred over red, yellow, orange, and other brighter, cheerier colors.

Coats and Jackets

Coats should include an unlined windbreaker, a lined windbreaker, and a parka of some sort, preferably with a hood. All should have shells made of some kind of water-repellent material. Sew pockets with rugged YKK zippers inside them for stashing extra gear. Coats with a snap-front that closes over a zipper are good because if the zipper breaks you still have a coat that you can close up.

Shirts

Shirts should include both long- and short-sleeved models, with most being long-sleeved (for versatility; you can always roll the sleeves up when it is hot). They should have extra buttons sewn in along the bottom front so that you always have them available. Try to skip cheap shirts that won't last long.

Headgear

Hats should consist of a plain ball cap and a wool skull cap at a minimum. The ball cap should have a full top—no mesh backs that let the wet in.

Trousers

Trousers should consist primarily of rugged jeans, but you would also be smart to have a pair or two of cotton chino-type trousers for hot weather. Sew military-style cargo pockets onto the outside of the legs for additional storage space.

Socks

Never skimp here. Get the best socks you can and take care of them by constantly rotating them (don't wear the same pair for more than a day) and washing them. Have different weights, too—enough to cover all seasons.

Footwear

Footwear should include good sneakers (but ones that appear dirty and stained, in keeping with your role) and a set of calf-high, insulated leather boots. For laces, use parachute (550) cord, which is very durable and versatile.

Gloves and Mittens

Gloves and mittens will probably be needed at some time regardless of where you are evading; even Miami can get chilly on January nights. A light pair of gloves and an insulated pair of mittens should suffice. The best material insofar as insulation goes is called Lamilite.

Underwear

Underwear is a personal choice for comfort and additional insulation. If you like it and don't mind the additional laundry, underwear should be of good quality and whatever style you prefer—boxers or briefs.

Belts

Every belt you have should be a money belt and be cut extra long with at least a foot of leather to spare in case you gain weight or need to use the belt to secure something other than your trousers. Always spread your money out in three or four hidden spots. Try not to carry it all at one time; hide it

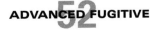

well if you stow it somewhere, and change the location frequently. (Don't pattern yourself when retrieving it.) Carrying large sums is always a risk, but sometimes a necessary one. Caution and paying attention to your surroundings are crucial.

Carrying Equipment

Since you will be staying on the move, never remaining in one area of town or a single location for more than a day, you will have to tote your gear around with you. If you are picturing yourself pushing around a shopping cart or some other wheeled transportation, I suggest you change the channel and picture yourself with a pack on your back. Granted, carts and the like do have their advantages, but any time you have to go inside a store or other such establishment you will likely find that you have to leave it outside. On the other hand, if you are wearing a pack you might easily be allowed to keep it on.

Packs

The pack you select should be just large enough to carry all your gear comfortably. Personal preference will dictate whether you select an internal or external frame model; each has advantages and disadvantages. Although I recommend a quality pack, if you buy it new you should dirty it up a little to fit in with your role. Remove brand names if possible; you wouldn't want to be trying to look like a down-and-out homeless wretch but be humping a state-of-the-art Kelty, Mountainsmith, or L.L. Bean expedition-sized pack. Wouldn't look kosher, eh? Try to go with as drab a color scheme as possible, or just dye it black.

A fanny pack to accompany your primary pack is a good idea for providing versatility, convenient access to frequently used items, and security for any cash, valuables, or essentials you carry.

Carts

If you do opt for a cart of some kind, make it fully securable; a bicycle chain lock will help. The traditional shopping cart isn't a very good choice insofar as durability and flexibility go, since their wheels break easily and they are difficult to push through snow. Then again, if snow is not a concern and you don't mind liberating a new cart from a shopping center's parking lot every time you need a new one, they can be all right. Should you decide to take one from a parking lot, do so at night and in the rain to minimize your being seen. I'm not advocating theft here, but when you're in a bad position you may have to do things that you normally wouldn't. Look at it this way: promise to make it up to the owner after your life gets back to normal, and then be true to your word.

Sustainment Equipment

This includes all the equipment in your pack that you will use to live your life, such as a stove, utensils, poncho, water bottles, and so on. It should only be used when you can't utilize the system's services and when it won't draw the attention of others who might think it peculiar that a homeless man has all kinds of genuine camping gear.

Stoves

Keep your stove selection simple and reliable. I recommend either an MSR XGK, which runs on almost any fuel, or a Peak 1 Apex II, which runs on either white gas or unleaded gas. Both are tough and easy to clean and service.

Sleeping Bags

Go with a bag filled with something other than down, since once down is wet it loses most of its heat-retaining ability. Synthetic filler like that used in quality bags like Wiggy's, Slumberjack, and Moonstone will serve you better anywhere rain is commonplace.

Lanterns and Flashlights

Go subtle with an L.L. Bean candle lantern or something akin to it.

Small, durable flashlights like the MiniMag are excellent and recommended. There really is no need to go with a large, heavy flashlight.

Ground (Sleeping) Pads

For comfort and reliability in ground pads, I recommend only one brand, Therm-A-Rest—preferably the Ultra Lite II model, which doesn't even weigh a pound.

Cooking Utensils

Go as light and rugged as possible and think small. Utensil sets with individual pieces that set inside the next larger piece are good for conserving space.

Working Knives

I strongly suggest a folding model with a locking blade (3 1/2 inches minimum) and some nice-to-have options like a bottle/can opener. Get one that is very unlikely to break on you and retains an edge well. Victorinox makes the best.

Shelter

I'd shy away from tents and opt for a couple of tarps or ponchos from which to build your own shelter with the aid of some ground stakes and a handful of bungee cords. A tent is just a bit too conspicuous.

USING MUNICIPAL SERVICES

The city will offer you certain survival services, such as shelters, places to eat, and health clinics. Regardless of the type of facility, use each only once in a rotating sequence. In other words, do not return to one facility until you have used all the others. This way you do not become a regular anywhere, which is just the way you want it.

Shelters

Shelters vary in size and security. The smaller shelters are generally safer in terms of the reduced number of potential thieves and assailants, but because there are fewer visitors, the staff and other homeless will remember you more easily should they be questioned. The opposite is true for large shelters, which are less secure but offer greater anonymity.

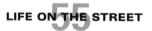
LIFE ON THE STREET

Regardless of the shelter, when you go to sleep secure your pack tightly and fasten it to you in some way, such as with a dark piece of cordage around your wrist tied at an unseen point on the pack. Dark cordage is more difficult to see at night (making it harder for the thief to detect) and by tying it to some unseen point on the pack you reduce the risk of the thief simply untying it. Attaching the pack to you at two different points (and using two different points on the pack) is an even better idea, since the thief may not suspect a backup alarm system.

Should you catch a thief in a shelter, leave immediately after warning him off as menacingly as possible. Do not raise a ruckus by calling the management—you will only draw more attention to yourself.

Approaching the clergy or nuns for shelter on an individual basis is risky because they will probably remember you.

Clinics and Hospitals

If you need medical attention and are ambulatory, seek a clinic that routinely services the homeless. They are used to riffraff like you and will often forget you.

If you find yourself being treated at an emergency room after being injured badly or knocked unconscious, be as vague as possible when answering questions about yourself. Give them just what they need and no more. If they ask about scars they find, do whatever you can to change the subject or make up a harmless, bland lie, i.e., don't say you got the scar in Vietnam, even if you did. The less they know about you the better off you'll be in the long run.

If cash is a problem, you can often get treatment for injuries or sicknesses that are not life threatening if you just put on the mentally ill act (not the dangerously mentally ill act, mind you, but the helpless, harmless mentally ill act). If they ask you to leave, don't. Just sit down or lie down and moan a lot. In the event that a security guard actually throws you out physically, lie right where he drops you. If you do this, most times they will come get you and treat you rather than call the cops, for fear of civil suits that might be brought against them for not treating you. If the cops do show up, stay with the act and leave when they say to. They are very unlikely to arrest you if you do this.

A fake ID can be helpful in cases where providing identification is a prerequisite of treatment.

Places To Eat

The proverbial soup kitchen or other homeless eatery is a place to get some food into your belly quickly but quietly and then leave without appearing to be in a hurry or any different from anyone else in there. Again, remember to rotate establishments. Also, keep a secret log of what you wore into each establishment the last time you were there, and then wear something different the next time.

America is a great country for giving away free food, drink, and entertainment. Start your day by sprucing yourself up, putting on a coat and tie, and heading to a major hotel with convention or large meeting facilities. Walk into the lobby and check out the activities placards for where what group is meeting when. For instance, the American Association of Food Retailers might be in the Ocean Room from 8:00 A.M. until 11:00 A.M. for an exhibit of new food merchandising displays. Many such groups and functions offer free food during these little get-togethers, and you are going to invite yourself.

From your bag of tricks whip out that blank name sticker that goes on your coat and scrawl some name on it, then walk right into the convention looking like you know what you're doing and you belong there. Head straight for the chow and fill a plate and grab a drink, then move to one of the displays but hang out just behind some other guys.

Keep eating as you politely listen to the guy running the display. As you begin to run out of food, go get some more and eat until you can't stand it anymore, then leave. If someone approaches you to make conversation, take the lead in the conversation by asking him who he's with and all about his job. Show a sincere interest in his work to keep him talking about himself and not you. If you feel the conversation is about to turn toward you, beg off by saying that you need to go to the bathroom or something.

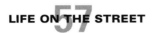

Time for dessert. Go to the mall or some other location where one of those frozen yogurt or ice cream stands with a million flavors is and appear puzzled as you ponder the menu. When asked what you would like, say you don't know because there's so much to choose from. Most such places offer samples for such people and love to pass them out for free. Try three or four, then casually disappear when the employee goes to serve someone else.

Now for a beer. In many cities in America, microbrews have taken over the market. Seattle, Washington, and Denver, Colorado, to name just two, are packed with microbreweries. Head into a bar and look over the fare. Ask for a sample, which most bars give out (note that some cities have more bars with free samples policies than others). Drink it, but even if you liked it say that you just don't care for it. Ask for another brand and drink that. Tell the barkeep that it's close but you're looking for something just a little different. Drink the third one, then get out of there.

Another idea is to check various bars for happy hour buffets, many of which are free. Yum.

CAMPING OUT

Where you will sleep when not in a shelter is a decision not to be made lightly. While park benches, steam grates, and the undersides of highway overpasses are the traditional digs, often such locales, when right in the city, will already be inhabited by plenty of other homeless people—and more are likely to show up after you arrive. This presents both a material security concern and a later identification concern. I recommend avoiding these places.

Instead, seek out park thickets, outlying overpasses, the backs of commercial support buildings with little foot and vehicle traffic, junkyards (whistle and call for the guard dogs before you enter; if they are there they will likely respond quickly), fire escapes on commercial buildings that are closed for the evening, and other such spots.

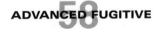

DEALING WITH THE AUTHORITIES

The time may come when you are forced to deal with the police in some way. If you are arrested and you have ever had your fingerprints taken—at just about any time by just about any organization—law enforcement will likely just feed the ones they take from you this time through the FBI's database for a match. The FBI computer doesn't make many mistakes, so you are almost assuredly going to be identified. Since there really aren't many viable means for having your fingerprints altered permanently that are available to people like us, the key is to not get arrested in the first place. If you develop your sense of awareness and use good judgment, you can almost always avoid being arrested by simply not doing or getting involved in things you shouldn't be doing or getting involved in.

However, you may be detained for any reason at any time and asked some questions, one of the first of which is likely to be what your name is followed by a demand for some identification. All your ID should be stowed in a secret compartment carefully sewn into the base of your pack (on the inside under all that weird stuff you have in there, which might consist of God knows what as far as the police are concerned) or elsewhere as long as it is a place viewed as a pain to get at by the police; never offer any ID, even a false ID, which is too easy for them to authenticate. If you suspect you will not be arrested but only detained and questioned on the spot for whatever reason, give a false name and stick to it. Answer questions with studied vagueness and deny all knowledge of whatever it is you are thought to have witnessed or heard. Stick to the story! Don't let them pressure you or sweat another story out of you. Be polite, but never give them any reason to think you might be of some use to them. Deny everything and admit nothing.

CHANGING CITIES

Travel by scheduled bus is one of the best means for changing cities. Get out there on the street and beg for money

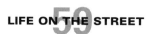

all day long until you have enough saved for a one-way trip to wherever it is you are heading, then pay cash up front for the ticket. Take a bus that leaves in the wee hours of the morning if possible; tired people don't remember as much as well-rested people do, and the more traveling you do at night, the better, for obvious reasons.

Don't talk with people on the bus. Sleep or pretend you are asleep as much as possible, but be aware of your surroundings and your gear. Never put any of your gear in the storage area beneath the bus—it can easily be stolen.

Hitching a ride can work, but do so subtly from a major truck stop rather than hitching along a highway or road. Many truckers are quite willing to share their cab for a while so long as you are clean, smell all right, and appear friendly, honest, and nonthreatening.

Finally, consider using existing trails such as the Appalachian Trail (AT) in the east (it runs from Georgia to Maine) or any of the many thousands of miles of maintained trails that crisscross the country. Maintaining your anonymity is simple on trails. Don't stop to chitchat with others; just say hello and keep on moving. When you make camp, do so well off the trail to avoid drawing the attention of the usually friendly backpackers who are sharing the trail with you. It is a common practice for many backpackers on trails to ask to pitch camp with you; they appear to automatically assume you are lonely and don't want you to be. Should someone start getting friendly and inquisitive, be gruff and cantankerous to ward them off. Two friends of mine, Bill and John, were on the AT several yards back when a lone hiker approached them in their camp. He was friendly and curious as most backpackers are, so Bill and John, when asked where they were from, responded gruffly, "Fuckin' Stratton," which is a small town in western Maine (and, no, they are not from Stratton). This response and their drinking lots of liquor and scowling helped the visitor to quickly make up his mind to camp elsewhere.

THE HIGHWAYMAN

"Highwayman" is the term used in Old England for those who robbed others on the road. But for our purposes a highwayman is a fugitive who lives on the road out of a vehicle of some kind.

There are definite advantages to living on the road as a vehicular vagabond of sorts, such as being able to stay on the move and therefore being harder to find. But as with any form of evasion, doing so requires some serious planning and thinking ahead with regard to things like how you are going to pay for the gas and upkeep on the vehicle, pay for food, and handle other expenses. You must also consider where you will spend most of your time traveling. Avoid the Northeast if you are from there, and so on. And always avoid Louisiana because the cops there will stop you for no reason and can even impound your vehicle and all your money without cause and keep part of what they impound! No, I'm not kidding.

Start by choosing a vehicle. Unless you are wealthy and have it arranged so that you will stay that way throughout your evasion, don't pick that Ned Sanders (Homer Simpson's saintly neighbor) type of recreational vehicle. Instead, buy a good used one that is just big enough for you. This way you don't spend as much on gas and the vehicle will be less memorable than one of those buildings on wheels.

Keep your vehicle in tip-top condition and always legal, although through the use of a complete name change (see the Paladin Press catalog for some excellent books on how to do this). Never speed or make other stupid mistakes on the road. Stay at the less popular RV parks, and if there's plenty of room, park as far away as possible from other campers. Stay inside as much as possible and don't answer the door if someone comes knocking; watch them as they leave. Always pay in cash, using bills with a normal worn appearance. Put some stickers from the major national parks on the back window, just like most other RVs have.

OVER THERE

Moving out of America and into a large city in some nation whose primary language is not English can be a daunting experience. Adapting to a different culture can range from being fairly painless to most trying. That's why you should have paid close attention in Chapter 2.

Regardless of what foreign country you move to, the indigenous people are going to know you are a foreigner as soon as you open your soup trap. And in many countries they'll know you aren't one of them as soon as they get a look at you. But there are ways of blending in that will make you less noticeable in certain countries.

As mentioned in Chapter 2, it helps to select a country that fits your general appearance. For instance, if you are of typically European stock, you should get to a country that has a lot people who look like you. If you have blond hair and blue

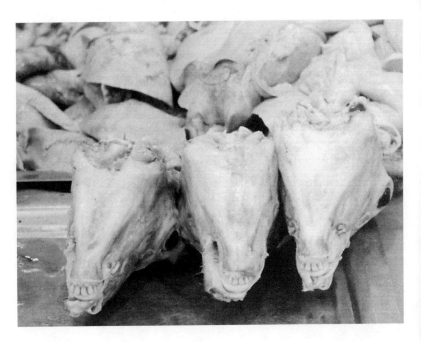

Eat what the natives eat.

eyes and are about six feet tall, you would fit in well in Scandinavia and Germany, but you would stick out like a black nun at a biker rally if you were to move to Taiwan.

Rent a travel video about the country you are considering going to and take note of the clothing styles worn there. If possible, have similar clothing on when you arrive. Have some currency of that country in your pockets, too, so you don't have to go to the currency exchange immediately. And have a plan for where it is in that country you want to go; don't wait until you get there to come up with a travel plan.

Eat what the natives eat and shop where they shop. Don't gawk or stare at things that people are buying to eat that disgust or shock you. When buying fish, check the eyes for clarity and the skin for springiness; if the eyes are dull or the skin dimples and stays that way, move on. (The earlier you arrive in the morning at the fish market, the fresher the fish in most cases. Beware of tricks like watering the fish with a hose

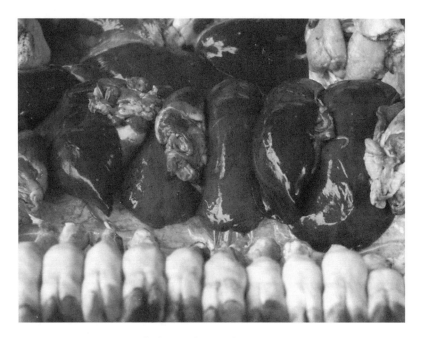

Don't turn your nose up at food items that repulse you.

to make them look fresher to the untrained eye.) Greet vendors first with the common greeting in their language and then politely ask them in another language you speak—yes, it could be English—if they speak that language. Even if they don't, they'll still figure out what you want and sell it to you.

When you are in public and you see some government officials coming your way or soldiers who might take an interest in you because you

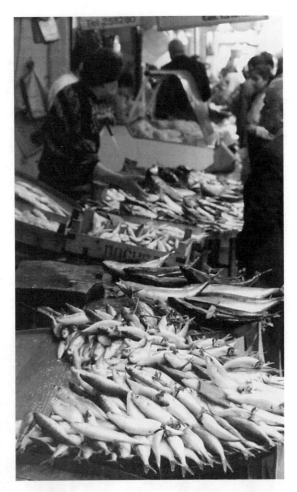

Is it fresh and safe?

are a foreigner, once they have seen you, do not try to avoid them by quickly ducking into a store or engaging a merchant in small talk. They'll see this as a ploy, and it will pique their interest. Walk right past them without making eye contact, as if you are no one special. This is nerve-racking but usually the most effective means of avoiding unwanted conversation.

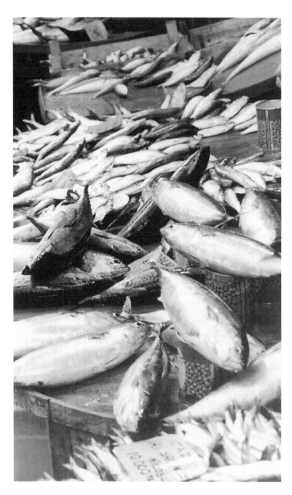
Check the eyes and skin, and it should smell fresh, not foul.

Consider carrying a false passport. Not a counterfeit passport, mind you, but a false passport. A false passport is legal in many countries (they will allow you to carry it but not use it going through customs) and can be bought from a vendor like Safeguard Services (1305 Grand Ave., #500, Nogales, AZ 85621). It is simply a replica of a passport once issued by a country that no longer exists, such as Rhodesia, British West Indies, New Hebrides, and British Guiana. A counterfeit passport is an illegally obtained genuine passport from a real country still in existence.

How you get to your new country is just as important as what you do after you get there. Most countries with multiple borders do not keep records of people who enter from a friendly neighboring state unless a visa is required. Avoid countries that require visas. In Europe it is remarkably easy to move from one country to the next with only so much as a cursory glance at your passport and perhaps a routine question or two about why you are entering that country (always answer that you are passing through on holiday to a country beyond that one), how long you intend to stay (just passing through or only a night), or what other countries you have visited recently (answer with countries

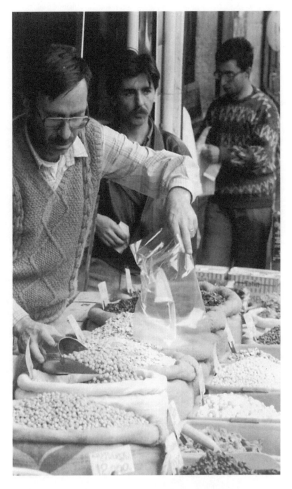

Don't speak the language? Point and shrug, and the merchant will figure a way to communicate with you.

that match the stamps in your passport, which should be friendly with the country you are now entering). Never carry firearms or explosives across international borders.

Trains, buses, and aircraft all go through customs checkpoints that see many tourists and have the most security. I recommend you opt for a less common entry and go for

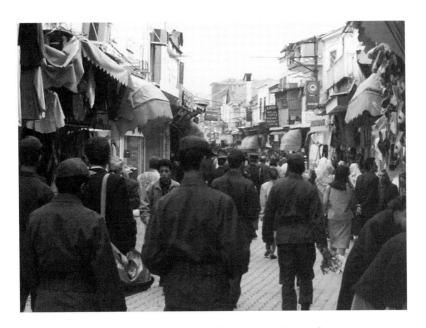

Are these soldiers looking for you? The fugitive constantly lives in fear.

something more subtle like arriving by having booked passage as a guest aboard a freighter. Many freighters and other cargo vessels accept passengers for a very modest fee, and it's 100-percent legal. Customs officials are often more lax when it comes to people at cargo shipping terminals.

Next up is a look at the rural fugitive.

PRIMITIVE PROSPECTS

The Wilderness Fugitive

"I sat on my log for days. By dusk on the first day I knew every detail of the landscape, the branches overhead, the mottled dying creeper in front of me, the midges dancing above the river, the shadows slowly moving around the tree-stump where the jeep-track came into view a hundred yards away in front. I knew the sounds: the jungle-sounds, the frog-sounds, the insect-sounds . . . I knew them much too well."

—Oliver Crawford
The Door Marked Malaya

No doubt you have heard of the legendary D.B. Cooper, the enterprising and daring bank robber who, with his loot strapped to his body, parachuted (Ooh-rah! Airborne!) out of a commandeered passenger jet somewhere over the Washington State wilderness, never to be seen or heard from again. Although I seriously doubt that, assuming he survived his jump and landing, he evaded for an extended period of time out there in the boonies, he did have to evade for a while before starting his new, richer life, wherever it is he started it. I wish I could have been a bird following him through the forest, watching every move and decision he made. (If by some fluke you are reading this, Mr. Cooper, I hope you will find a way to drop me a line safely. Your evasion experiences would make great reference material.)

The decision to conduct your evasion in a wilderness area is one that requires much forethought, planning, and training—more than that needed for urban evasion because of the nonexistence of support structures provided by the government and kind people who don't mind giving out handouts. You will have to rely on only your wits, training, and equipment to survive and evade those who wish to do you harm in some way.

Let's be right up front here. If you think wilderness evasion is romantic and adventuresome in a Hollywood sort of way, you are very, very mistaken. There is nothing amusing, fun, or desirable about hiding like an animal for a long period of time—months to years—from armed men who are hunting you with the intent to either capture or kill you. You are not in Hollywood, and this isn't a *project* being filmed *on location*. Understand that right now. I have lived like an animal in miserable places and hidden from people who would have liked very much to have found me. Looking back on it, no, I wouldn't trade those experiences for all the proverbial tea in China, but I also remember the terrible fear and angst that lived in my guts as I tried desperately to remain undetected. It's a feeling I hope you never experience for yourself. And I remember the freezing nights, unbelievable heat, and cold steel rain that at times seemed to never end. I remember the gnawing hunger and raw thirst, the cruel insects, and the mind-numbing pain of crippling injuries.

Sound like a good time to you?

Nevertheless, wilderness evasion is an option with definite advantages for certain fugitives, but know that those fugitives must be cut from a certain cloth and have the stuff—the determination, resourcefulness, knowledge, and skills—to undertake the most demanding and extreme form of evasion there is. The wilds of this planet can be most inhospitable—as can many of the people on it—and you must be mentally, spiritually, and physically prepared to tough it out for a long time under the most severe conditions. Wilderness evasion is not for the undisciplined, misguided, or weak. Nature plays by one set of rules, Hers, and She doesn't take kindly to fools, idiots, and crybabies.

That said, let's study what it takes to become truly prepared for wilderness evasion.

REQUIRED SKILLS FOR THE ULTIMATE TEST

First of all, if you think reading this book and some great camping gear is all you need to prepare yourself for wilderness evasion, you are sadly mistaken. The backwoods fugitive who successfully evades those who seek him is always someone who has not only read everything about the craft of backwoods evasion but who has spent countless hours applying and practicing the skills he read about. Some good books and a positive attitude aren't enough to keep you free. You must *read*, *study*, *comprehend*, and then *do*—again and again until each skill becomes instinctive—in order to reach the level of evasion acuity necessary for safe and effective wilderness evasion. We must start with basic wilderness skills.

Firecraft

Forget all those beautiful, friendly fires you enjoyed while on camping trips with your family or backpacking or hunting trips with your buddies. Every fire you build from here on out will be underground or otherwise completely shielded from in-range human eyes, regardless of who those eyes belong to.

The Makings of a Fire

Fire is a chemical reaction requiring three components: fuel, oxygen, and heat. The fuel can be anything combustible that the wilderness fugitive has available, ranging from *punk wood* (the wood found inside a partially rotten long) and *squaw wood* (the brittle lower branches of conifers like pine, spruce, and fir, also called Indian kerosene) to grass, leaves, sticks, branches, gasoline, cotton, fire paste, and so on. Oxygen—air—must be available, and the fugitive can use his own breath to coax a fire or the air provided by nature in the form of a breeze or even still air. The heat source refers to not only

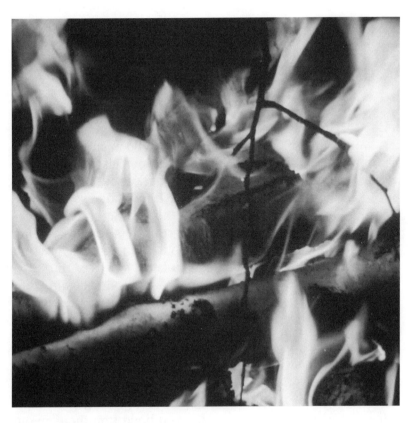

Open campfires are taboo.

the initial spark or flame applied to the lower echelon of fuel, tinder, but also to the flames of the fire itself. If at any time any one of these three components is removed, even for the briefest of moments, the fire will be extinguished instantly. These three components are what are commonly known as the *fire triangle*.

Starting any fire, but especially an evasion fire, requires forethought and planning. You must gather or otherwise come up with the three levels of fuel you will need for your evasion fire. These are tinder, kindling, and the main fuel itself.

Tinder is the first level of fuel you will use when getting your fire going. It must be very dry and easily ignitable with the faintest of sparks or flame. Tinder might consist of any of the following:

- the downy fiber from a cattail, thistle, or milkweed seed head
- nests of rodents and birds (beware of bird mites and ticks in these nests)
- pocket lint
- tiny tufts of cotton or wool fiber from a shirt
- cotton balls from your fire kit (kept in a small watertight container; the cotton can be lightly coated with petroleum jelly for added burn time)
- pitch powder; this is the powdery residue you scrape off spruce, fir, or pine pitch
- charred cotton
- crumbled, dried animal dung from a herbivorous animal (moose, bison, caribou, etc.)
- the thinnest possible shavings from dry conifer wood
- the bark of a paper or yellow birch
- tufts of dead grass or sedges
- a pulled-apart piece of steel wool from your fire kit
- extremely thin shavings from a tinder polypore mushroom

Experiment with potential tinder long before you start your evasion. This way you won't be wasting your time and energy when you really don't have either to waste.

Once your tinder is burning well, slowly add some kindling at a rate that

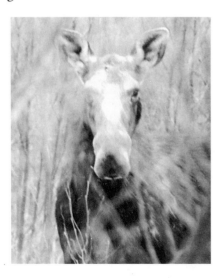

Dry moose droppings make good tinder.

PRIMITIVE PROSPECTS

allows it to catch without choking the fire's oxygen supply. Remember that each level of fuel requires all three parts of the fire triangle at all times—don't rush the fire.

Kindling includes the following:

- twigs about as thick as a pencil; always use the driest hardwood twigs you can find to lessen smoke output
- midsize shavings from a tinder polypore mushroom
- fairly thick shavings from a dead hardwood branch
- the innermost portion of a dead hardwood log (punk wood)

If you are unsure whether a certain piece of potential kindling will burn with little smoke, cut or break off a tiny piece and try it.

The heaviest of main fuel should be no thicker than your little finger or so. You might be surprised to find how hot and useful a fire you can build with the right main fuel of this size. Main fuel includes the following:

- dead hardwood sticks
- thick hardwood shavings (see the aforementioned description of maximum thickness)
- appropriately thick shavings from a tinder polypore mushroom

By removing the bark from all fuel, you will reduce the amount of smoke the fire generates.

Fire Site Selection and Preparation

This is often an easy task when you are not concerned with being detected, but it can be tough as a survivor until you get the hang of things. Remember that you will not be building fires in the open, which means every fire must be secretive. This is so important a concept that I want to stress it one more time: *Do not build any fire anywhere that exposes the flames or smoke to detection. To do so puts you at tremendous risk.*

Although the Dakota hole is certainly the preferred fire lay for the wilderness fugitive, it may not be feasible or absolutely necessary all the time. However, any nocturnal fire built anywhere but in some subterranean location like a cave, grotto, or abandoned mine shaft (and you might be surprised how many abandoned mine shafts there are in some parts of North America, especially in the Mojave Desert's Bullion range) should be a Dakota hole. This excludes, of course, fires you build in old trappers' cabins and other remote structures you might use from time to time. (As always, you must leave no trace of your having been there when you leave, and still, this is a risky proposition unless you are sure the owner is long dead or will otherwise not be returning any time soon and the chances of someone else stumbling upon the cabin are extremely remote.)

Daytime fires kept very small and set in dense thickets—with trees tall enough to fully diffuse the smoke before it disappears as no more than wisps above the canopy—are acceptable provided you feel quite sure the smoke will not be

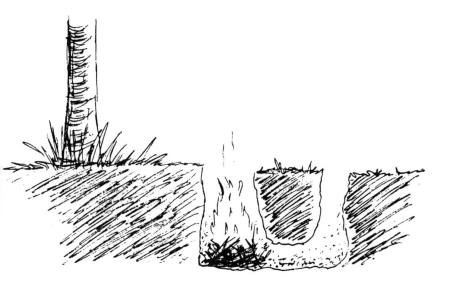

Dakota hole.

detected by anyone from a vantage point above the thicket, such as an aircraft or terrain feature. As with any evasion fire, the flames must be kept small, and only the driest hardwood twigs and very small sticks with the bark removed can be used.

The precise location on the ground where you lay your fire is crucial. The most dense and seemingly impenetrable part of the thicket—so thick that no one can see anything going on where you are inside—is where you want to put your fire. The fire should be set surrounded by logs to further mask the flames, and on windy days you must consider the possibility that someone might smell the smoke. (In this case no fire should be set there or anywhere. Also, if you feel those hunting you might have thermal imaging equipment, never build a fire in the area in which you suspect them to be.)

In snow country, beware of boughs above the fire you have set at the base of trees—especially conifers—that hold snow. The little warmth from the flames may be enough to melt the snow and send it crashing down onto the fire, snuffing it out instantly. Shake the branches softly first to rid them of the snow they hold.

After gathering all the materials you will need to start, foster, and propagate the fire, clear the ground where you will set the fire of any material that may burn, but which you do not want to burn. Leaves, grass, twigs, and other things that might catch fire must be set aside well out of the reach of the flames.

By removing the top half inch or so of soil and detritus from the fire site and placing it aside, you will have natural material at hand that you can use for concealing the fire site when you depart. (Remember that this is a fire no more than a foot in diameter, so there won't be that much dirt and detritus in the first place.) Take note of the ground's appearance before you remove it so you can replace it as realistically as possible. If the ground is snow-covered, it won't do to replace the snow you remove with the same snow, since it will appear disturbed by including bits of vegetation and possibly soil. Instead, from a site some distance away from the fire site, gather some snow from branches and the very top of the snow pack—being care-

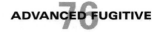

ful not to disturb either enough to give away your ruse—for covering the fire site before you leave. I like to look for dead, standing trees (*snags*) to build a fire beside so that I can push the snag down onto the fire site, thus covering it in a natural manner, when I am ready to leave. I then make sure I wipe out all my tracks as I move on. Don't build the fire so close to the tree that the flames scorch the trunk—an attentive tracker will see the blackened streaks and know you were there.

Water Procurement and Preparation

Hopefully you will have selected an evasion area that offers plenty of water in all four seasons. The desert is seldom your best bet for evasion and survival.

Locating Water Sources

To find water, first study your topographic map. Note not only the locations of obvious water sources like lakes, ponds, rivers, streams, springs, and creeks but also the following:

- draws
- intermittent (seasonal) streams
- arroyos
- gulches
- cliff bases
- small patches of green on the map surrounded by beige or brown, illustrating the presence of living vegetation in dry areas (these mean water is available probably a short way below the surface)
- valley floors

The wilderness fugitive can also be watchful for signs given by nature that water is nearby or lying in a certain direction, such as the following:

- the sound of frogs at night and just before dawn
- birds such as doves flying at dusk and dawn in a particular direction
- the call of the cactus wren if you are in the American

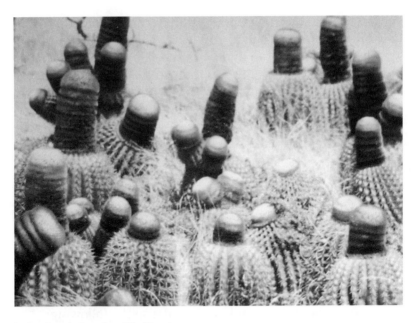

Many barrel-shaped cacti hold water.

Southwest (the cactus wren's call is a *chuh-chuh-chuh-chuh*, and the bird likes mesas and sunny hillsides with thorn trees and cacti in abundance; it is seldom far from a water source)
- converging game trails—follow the single trail two convergent trails form; the single trail will often lead to a water source
- the outside edges of bends on dry streambeds hold water as little as a foot down
- vines; many hold water
- cacti; cutting open cacti like the pincushion or barrel cactus will yield water in the pulp
- cattle, horses, bison, and pronghorn in open range land all walking in a column; this usually means they are moving toward a water source
- insects hovering over a certain spot; it might be a dead critter, or it might be a seepage or puddle

- game trails used by elk are heavily trodden; the trail may lead to a wallow
- an osprey; this fish hawk is always near water
- a bald eagle; the bald eagle frequently grabs fish from lakes and rivers
- waterfowl circling in the late afternoon or early morning indicate water they are considering landing in
- wading birds such as herons, bitterns, and egrets are never far from water; watch where they fly to

Collecting Water

The wilderness fugitive must always be ready to collect dew and rainwater at the following opportune times:

- in the morning when a dew is on the ground (wrap absorbent cloth around each ankle and walk through the vegetation, then wring out the cloth into a container)
- during periods of rain (set out small containers to catch the runoff; also, after a rain you can wrap those

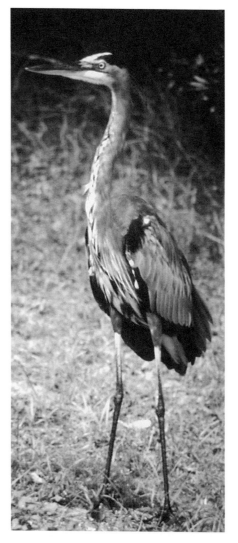

The blue heron is always near water.

PRIMITIVE PROSPECTS

absorbent cloths around your arms and legs and walk through thick vegetation to gather the rain dripping off of it)

Purifying Water

Although there is no real need to purify rainwater that has just fallen and that has been collected off vegetation that isn't toxic, the fugitive must purify all other water in order to eliminate or at least greatly reduce the chances of inadvertent poisoning by natural or manmade contaminants. Whereas it is obviously inadvisable to drink any water from a source that has dead animals lying around it, all water, no matter how clear and odorless and regardless of the fact that it came from a running stream high in the mountains, must be purified in some way. This is because natural pathogens like *Giardia lamblia* and *Campylobacter jejuni* are often found in what appears to be a pristine mountain stream.

There are three primary means of water purification for the wilderness fugitive: boiling, chemical purification, and filtration.

Boiling. This will kill all natural contaminants like cryptosporidia, *Campylobacter jejuni*, cholera, typhoid, fecal coliform bacteria, *Giardia lamblia*, *E. coli*, salmonella, and parasites; however, it may not have any effect on manmade toxins. Bring the water to a rolling boil for a few minutes, and every natural contaminant will die.

Chemicals. This means iodine and chlorine. The wilderness fugitive should have an ample supply available. Follow the directions on the bottle—you may need more chemical for cloudy or cold water. Note that some manmade toxins will not be neutralized by these chemicals.

Filtration. There are a number of good filters on the market, but the best is one made by General Ecology (151 Sheree Blvd., Exton, PA 19341)—the First Need filter. This filter removes darn near everything, natural or manmade. To rid

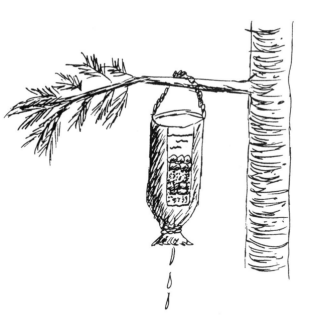

Trouser leg filter.

water of suspended particulate matter prior to purification (don't confuse the two; filtering water in order to remove suspended matter isn't the same as filtering out toxins), use a trouser leg filter (see the illustration).

Water is critical to your survival, and you should never underestimate your body's need for it. Even in cold climates your body uses large amounts of water. Three or four quarts a day is considered the minimum in a temperate zone while performing light work. Adjust accordingly.

If you are thirsty, drink. Thirst is your body's way of telling your brain that water is required. Rationing water is senseless—it does no good in your canteen. When you drink until you are no longer thirsty, your body can store the extra water for later use—the body doesn't waste water it doesn't use immediately. Dark urine, nausea, and a nagging headache are three signs of dehydration.

Food Procurement

Much of your time is going to be spent trying to acquire food. The fugitive who forages for plants and mushrooms, depends on fish a great deal (in areas with fish), and keeps an eye out for small game while always being ready for big game

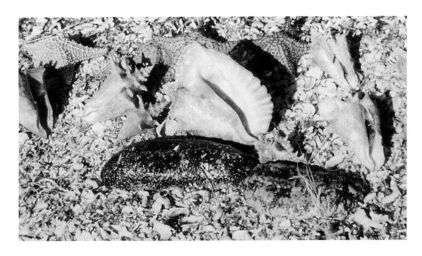
Sea cucumbers and conchs make for good eating.

(if the situation suddenly presents itself and you are confident not only that no one is around or searching for you in the area but that you can avoid leaving any sign of the big game—deer, moose, caribou, bear—being killed and cleaned thereabouts) is a fugitive who stands a better chance of making it than the guy who dwells solely on one type of food. If the fugitive learns to ignore cultural food biases against insects and amphibians, all the better.

Hunting

It might be a good idea to become proficient with silent primitive weapons if you have reason to believe that the sound of a firearm discharging might draw unwanted attention your way. Atlatls, slingshots, boomerangs, archery equipment, and blowguns, are all options, but using them effectively requires lots of practice. If you want to become proficient fairly quickly with a silent primitive weapon, I highly recommend *Blowguns: The Breath of Death* (Paladin Press).

If noise is not an immediate consideration, however, firearms are still your best bet for putting food on your plate.

Hunting firearm selection for the fugitive is dictated by the species of game in the evasion area. Generally speaking, if the fugitive expects to take the occasional big game species such as elk or moose and feed off the prepared (smoked and airdried) meat for months rather than taking small game on a regular basis, then a bolt-action, scoped rifle in an appropriate caliber is called for. These include .30-06 Springfield, .300 Winchester Magnum, .300 Weatherby Magnum, and .338 Winchester Magnum; such calibers have tremendous takedown capability. Bolt-action rifles manufactured by companies like Remington, Sako, Sauer, Winchester, Ruger, and Weatherby are more accurate than autoloaders, pumps, and lever-actions, and they have far fewer malfunctions. A quality scope on top of the rifle should have excellent light-gathering ability for shooting situations in dim light (dusk and dawn), be rugged and absolutely fog-proof, be easily adjustable, and offer variable power such as 3X-9X or something close to that. The Redfield Golden Five Star, Nikon Monarch UCC, Weaver V-9, Bausch & Lomb Elite 4000, Pentax Lightseeker II, and Leupold Vari-X II are outstanding.

If small game such as rabbits and hares, rodents (woodchuck, muskrat, beaver, squirrel, marmot), birds, and the like are going to be the norm, a smaller-caliber rifle is needed. The .223 Remington, .22-250 Remington, and 6mm Remington are good choices. The same action and scope advice applies. Avoid the diminutive .22 as your only weapon; it is not powerful or versatile enough for anything but fairly close shots at small game. Since you aren't hunting for sport but rather for survival, skip the shotgun as a primary hunting weapon and plan on taking just about all of your game before it tries to escape or even knows you're there. This means that birds sportsmen fire at on the wing will now be taken while they are still on the ground (or water) milling about or sitting in a tree. Suppose you are evading in a region where many waterfowl exist. In that case, a shotgun would be advisable because it can be used to sluice a flock while it rests on the surface, resulting in several ducks or geese being killed rather than only one.

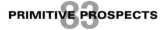

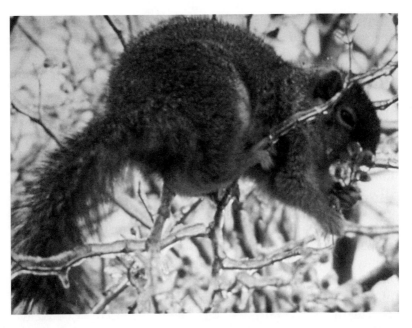

When squirrels are feeding, the fugitive can often get very close. (Photo courtesy of U.S. Fish & Wildlife Service)

You must also consider the logistics of resupplying your stock of ammunition. This can be done by reloading your own as it is needed, buying it as needed, or caching it. Reloading requires special equipment that is bulky and will make the fugitive less mobile, but it is an option in regions where you expect to stay holed up in one location for a good bit of time. Buying it means you are going to have to come into contact with other people and therefore risk capture. This leaves caching, which is by far the best choice. (Check out *State-of-the-Art Survival Caching*, a video from Paladin Press.)

Fishing

Fish should be a high priority in most evasion situations in the wild. They are easy for the fugitive to catch without drawing attention to himself or his whereabouts. Simple fishing sets that are known to you but go unnoticed by others are

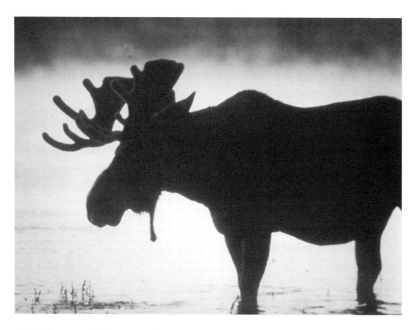

The bull moose calls for a powerful round. (Photo courtesy of U.S. Fish & Wildlife Service)

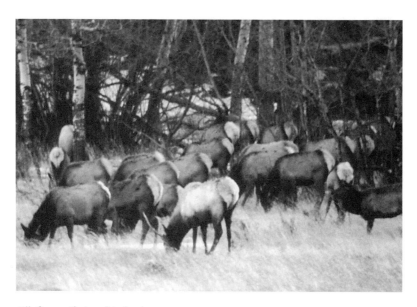

Elk frequently travel in herds.

very effective and worth your time and effort, and a gill net can easily be made and used surreptitiously.

The gill net is set in water preferably containing fish that roam about. The size of the mesh is determined by the size of the fish you wish to catch. Set it so that none of the net can be seen from the bank. You can do this by rigging the net to two poles jammed into the bottom so that they don't stick above the surface. Mark the spot somehow with a subtle sign along the bank adjacent to the set. Check it once every 24 hours or so unless the water is really teeming with fish, and check it only at night to reduce the risk of detection further.

The hoop set is also an excellent evasion net, provided you keep the set hidden. It uses the lobster/crab trap principle of allowing something to enter but not to leave. The illustration shows how simple it is. I have used these nets in such places as the bayous of Louisiana and had great success.

An easy way to use fishing line (20-pound test is a good tensile strength) and a hook is to skewer some bait on the very sharp, barbed hook, preferably a treble hook, and toss the bait

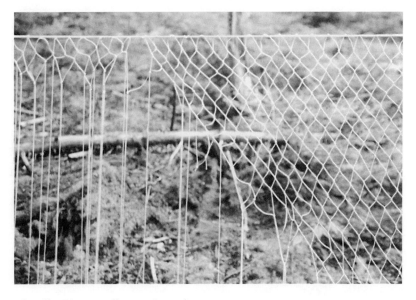

The gill net is an excellent evasion tool.

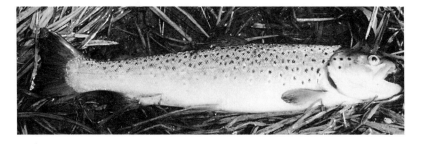

Fish are vulnerable to many ploys.

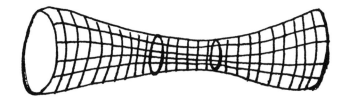

Hoop net.

in the water with a small lead weight (sinker). Tie the other end of the line to a bush or branch underwater. Check it from time to time, again, at night.

I don't recommend electrocution for fishing in most cases because it's too easy for dead fish to drift away, and you run the risk of their being seen by someone looking for you. However, in very small backwaters and in tide pools it can be useful. Get yourself a hand-held crank generator and some wire and run the wire down into the water. Crank away. The stunned fish will float up. Scarf 'em up.

Don't use explosives to fish. Noise aside, they muddy the water, and muddy water is evidence of you. Besides, you could end up like the idiot cop in Medway, Maine, who recently rigged a charge to fish with and had the thing blow off part of his hand. This is bad for morale and not too good for your career, either.

Trapping

Traps and snares, if set in a way that does not draw the attention of other humans, can be highly effective and I recommend them. One of the best evasion snares is the drag snare. It allows the game to break free of the anchor and thus not die where it was caught, but arranges for the game to become caught up in brush away from the anchor set and remain alive and well until found and dispatched by you. The game sticks its head through the loop and the loop tightens as the game moves forward. When the game panics the drag stick breaks free of the anchor set and the game scampers off, dragging the stick, which will soon become snagged in a bush or something and hold the animal in place. The fugitive comes along and checks the set, sees that it has been sprung, and then begins a concentric outward circle search for the critter. He finds the beast and kills it, then resets the snare.

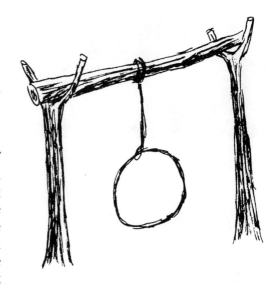

Drag snare.

Foraging Plants

The number and variety of edible plants in North America, let alone the world, is truly astounding. Okay, so there's a downside, too—there are also plenty of plants out there that, if eaten, will drop you in your tracks like a .338 Winchester Magnum drops a prairie dog at 100 yards. You get

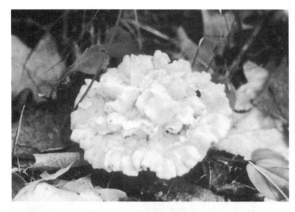

The chicken mushroom or sulfur shelf is a fine edible.

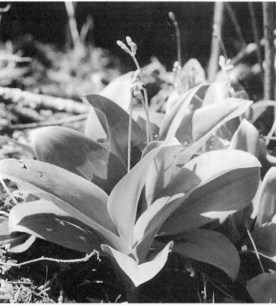

False hellebore contains a nasty cardiotoxin.

Labrador tea grows in alpine areas.

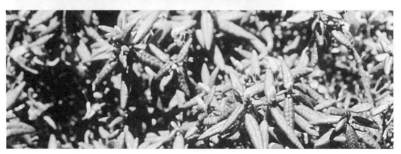

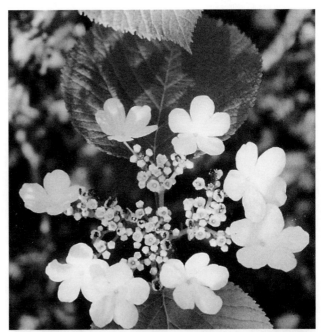

The hobble-bush has tasty berries.

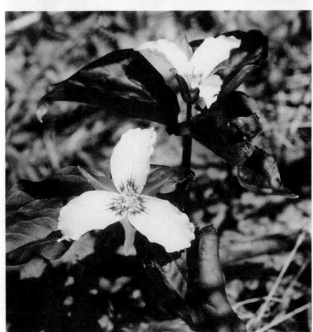

Trilliums are good when they are young (before they bloom).

ADVANCED FUGITIVE

the picture. But the wilderness survivor can easily—make that *very* easily—learn to identify edible, nutritious plants and prepare them for eating. Look at it this way: when you stroll through the produce section of your local supermarket, can you identify most of the veggies therein? You can? Then you can learn to identify the edible produce growing in your evasion area. There's no hocus-pocus, no Tom Brown "Tracker" bush- or tree-spirit worshipping—none of that crap. (As a matter of fact, forget all that communing-with-nature, tree-hugging stuff. It might get you dead.) It's simply a matter of attention to detail and using your gray matter to remember things.

The first step is to find out what edible and toxic plants are available in the region in which you are considering evading. When performing your evasion area evaluation, identify as many plants as possible by using a good reference on the subject (see Appendix G). If there aren't at least 20 edible plant species available and abundant spring through fall, and half a dozen or so during the winter months (in snow climates), you may want to consider another area.

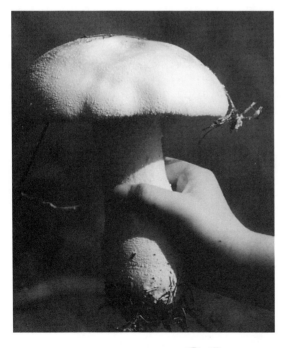

Is it a delicious and safe horse mushroom or a deadly amanita? Something altogether different? You'd better know before eating it.

I think it is very important to have an outstanding knowledge of which plants and mushrooms are edible and which are not before you take up residence in an area. As a fugitive you shouldn't be having to run taste tests on flora and fungi you find and hope are edible. Have the knowledge *before* you begin your evasion.

Foraging can be as simple as you make it when it comes to plants and mushrooms. A while back I was hiking through the woods with a bunch of people when we stopped for a break. While they sat there and drank water, I looked about at the local flora. Within 20 feet of us were blackberries (which I gorged myself on), wood sorrel, plantain, assorted grasses and oaks, clover, a chicken mushroom, watercress, Queen Anne's lace, and arrowhead, all of which are highly edible in some way. Mixed in amongst these were two species of nasty amanita mushrooms, poison ivy, an eastern diamondback rattlesnake, and water hemlock, all of which can really screw up your karma.

Finding Shelter

Although I am bigger than average, I managed to squeeze into this tiny cave in New England that had been formed by two granite boulders and erosion between them. Sure, it was tight in there (I couldn't stretch out), but remember that you are not camping—you are evading. As my friend John says when he teaches advanced evasion techniques to those who need to know, "You can't be a slave to comfort and expect to stay free."

Cabins and Other Standing Structures

Wilderness evasion shelters come in all shapes and sizes and materials. Although you might get away with staying in a remote, hidden cabin of some kind for some time, this kind of luxury won't often be available, but might be depending on the circumstances. John and I have stayed in a tiny cabin overlooking a remote valley and felt confident that no one would surprise us there, because even those few people who had been to the cabin before often had a hard time finding it again because of the trees and terrain that surround it. In the

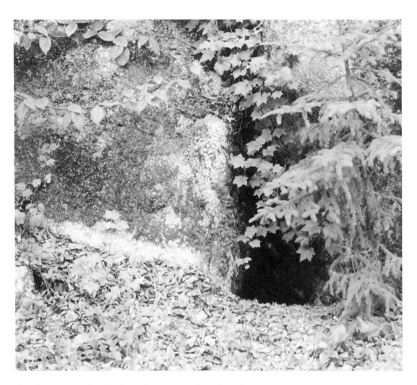

Small caves are less likely to be known about by others.

summer the forest hid the cabin well, and in winter the deep snows and steep terrain were too daunting for all but the most insistent woodsmen.

Other cabins (such as the 10th Mountain Division cabins in the Rockies) and structures (such as the lean-tos along the Appalachian Trail that are maintained by the Appalachian Trail Club) can be used, although other people passing through will definitely show up. The trick is to make it appear as if you just arrived for an overnight stay, and that you aren't a fugitive at all but a hiker. There are many such shelters in national parks and along popular hiking trails. Yes, using them is risky. However, they are an option if you are absolutely certain that no one is looking for you in that area and that you can make anyone believe you are just another hiker. To do this you must keep firearms out of sight (hide them outside) and have a false ID (read one of Paladin Press's new ID books, such as *The Paper Trip I & II, The Real World of Alternate ID Acquisition, New I.D. in America, The Heavy Duty New Identity,* and *Reborn in the USA*). Keep that ID in your gear in case someone should search it when you aren't looking, and have a full, practiced cover story to go with it when asked who you are, what you do, and so on. Keep only what a normal hiker would have with him inside the shelter and the rest of your heavy-duty survival supplies outside and hidden.

Using someone's private cabin is more risky for the most part because you just don't know if the owners are going to show up there while you are in it. I recommend only using such a cabin under the following circumstances: 1) if it is extremely remote, 2) if the weather is very bad (deep snows and very cold temps), and 3) if you will be able to see them coming in time enough for you to get out without being seen or otherwise detected. This means that you are going to have to stay ready to run at a moment's notice. Keep everything packed that you aren't using at the moment and be ready to brush out your tracks.

Abandoned mines are a possibility, although most are sealed in some way. Most mines have a single primary entrance and at least two escape exits, so check the area for the latter if the primary is sealed. Also, check the area for signs of recent human activity—footprints, tire tracks, beer cans, fire rings, and so on. You can find mines on topographic maps.

Natural Shelters

Like the aforementioned tiny cave, natural shelters are frequently less than cozy, but sometimes they can be great. These are the shelters you use when you suspect someone may be in the area looking for you and when the situation otherwise dictates that you need a shelter and fast.

While caves can be nice, how many times have you actually run across them by accident? Not many, if any, I'd bet. The thing is that some areas have lots of caves (Kentucky, Tennessee,

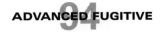

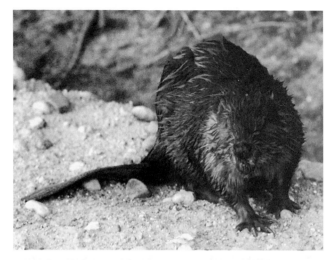

The beaver won't want to give up his home.

Beaver lodges are good evasion hides.

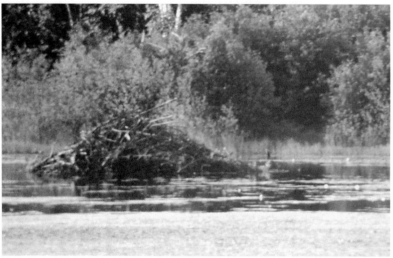

Arkansas) but most of them are well known and used regularly by spelunkers and children. Caves are also often watery and cold.

Rock overhangs, blow-downs (trees that have been felled by acts of nature), and hollow logs (or logs that can be easily hollowed out because they are rotten inside) are all frequently available to the fugitive. One of the simplest evasion shelters you can rig is one consisting of a blow-down in a thicket with a poncho or tarp draped over it to form a tent. Secure the sides with brush and other material to disguise the shelter. Eliminate your tracks leading into the thicket and set detours along the natural avenues of approach into the thicket. This can be done by arranging other blow-downs in a natural appearance across these avenues, thereby casually forcing other humans to go around you; the idea is to make it just hard enough so that they head away from your secret shelter without it appearing that someone intentionally put that detour there.

Beavers have made a big comeback since the fur market declined and trapping fell out of favor with the kinder, gentler folk, but this is to your advantage. Beavers build shelters called lodges, which have underwater entrances often big enough for a man to get through. To find the entrance just watch the primary approach route of the beavers as they swim toward the lodge, which is a large mound of sticks, branches, and mud. Most of the time the beaver will swim in a straight line right for the entrance. Make about a four-foot spear and take it underwater with you, along with a large knife. Find the entrance and surface with the spear ready to fend off the mad beaver(s) the moment you break the surface. Adult beavers will usually defend their property, but they can be killed or chased off if you are aggressive and very menacing. Watch those teeth and claws. Once they are dead or gone, retrieve your gear and return to the lodge for use as a temporary/emergency hide. Use some of the branches and sticks from the inside of the lodge to seal the entrance from the inside so that you'll hear the beaver if he tries to get back in.

Don't use gator hibernation holes; too risky.

Keep in mind that any natural shelter that looks good to you also looks good to wildlife. Bears, mountain lions, snakes, insects, bats, opossums, raccoons, and other creatures may have to be asked to leave the premises.

Constructed Evasion Shelters

These are shelters you build from scratch.

In *Fugitive: How to Run, Hide, and Survive,* I discussed the

U.S. military's formula for building evasion shelters, BLISSS—which stands for blend in, low in silhouette, irregular in shape, small, survivable, and secluded. Every evasion shelter you build must abide by this formula if you have to avoid all human contact. In case you haven't read that book (and I am very disappointed in you if you haven't), let's go over the formula here.

B—*Blend in.* This means camouflage to the extreme. The fugitive must make the evasion shelter appear to be just another piece of the environment and be totally unremarkable. Every step must be taken to eliminate any feature of the hide that draws attention.

L—*Low in silhouette.* The lower to the ground, the better. In fact, some excellent hides can be made entirely or partially underground. The human eye, unless trained with the owner's brain to search for hides low to the ground, looks for things at about eye level.

I—*Irregular in shape.* Think about the shapes in most environments. They are varied in some ways (blow-downs, etc.) but constant in others (standing trees). The human eye is naturally attracted to anything that seems out of place, so the evasion shelter should be shaped to avoid attention.

S—*Small.* Make your shelter just big enough for you and whatever you have with you (never leave anything outside the shelter, even for a moment). However, the shelter must be large enough for you to get some rest.

S—*Survivable.* When I teach a course on evasion I often find that people forget to build the hide with survivability in mind. You must build for a worst-case scenario each and every time. Never assume that nice weather is going to stay that way. In many climates, like the mountains and desert, daytime temps can easily be in the 90s, but once night falls they drop into the 40s. A shelter built for the 90s doesn't work well in the 40s.

S—*Secluded.* Build as far away from trails and roads as possible, preferably in a swamp, pocosin, or thicket, or in terrain that is intimidating and taxing. Make it hard for someone to come look for you—so hard that they convince themselves that there's no way you can be back in there because it's just too hard to get to.

The natural materials you use when building your hide must be taken without leaving obvious evidence. Branches and logs picked up off the ground usually leave impressions in the ground, and everyone knows they don't get up and walk off by themselves. Moss peeled off a rock or log will leave a dark spot that gets unneeded attention. Limbs torn off trees that don't end up on the ground beneath the tree get attention, too. This is why building your hide in as intimidating a place as possible is very wise: if there's no one there to see what you have used, you have less to worry about.

Navigation

If you are going to be out in the boonies, your navigation skills must be outstanding. Entire books on navigation are available, and I recommend you study one like *Wilderness Wayfinding* from Paladin Press.

Navigation for the fugitive requires skills in map and compass work, yes, but goes miles beyond that. Being able to triangulate to determine your location, shoot an intersection to locate a certain feature on the map, plot bearings and run legs, determine slope, recognize terrain features, and so on are only the beginning when it comes to evasion navigation. The fugitive must also be expert at primitive navigation techniques like celestial navigation and terrain association and be very good at using the land's natural features to aid him in getting around. And if you have an instinctive ability to navigate (known in the trade as woodsense), all the better.

To learn navigation in an instructional environment, check out your local college or contact your local orienteering club. There are a few organizations that teach land nav for a fee, and some are well worth it. Get a catalog before sending your money so that you don't end up wasting your time at a tree-hugger school, unless that's what you're into.

Medical Skills

A course in basic first aid is not enough. The wilderness

fugitive must be skilled at least to the Emergency Medical Technician (EMT) level if he wants to stand the best chance of surviving his evasion. The American Red Cross, local hospital, and college are good places to start your training in emergency medicine, but don't stop there. You are going to need experience in primitive medicine, too. Read *Ditch Medicine* and *Survivalist's Medicine Chest*, both from Paladin Press.

Herbal medicine is also a topic that is important to the fugitive. Many colleges now offer courses in this art and science, and there is a growing interest in it across the country. Many of the pharmaceutical products we enjoy today were developed from plants, and herbal medicine is quite a bit simpler to learn and practice than you might think. It can be as simple as curing your upper respiratory infection (URI) by inhaling the steam from a pot of boiling cedar twigs.

Coexisting with Dangerous Animals

Before we move along, some common-sense guidance on encounters with dangerous animals that all too often tends to be forgotten at the wrong time and in the wrong place.

Avoidance is the word of the day here, and the best way to avoid problems with wild animals is to learn where they live and what they (and their sign) look like. For instance, in depression meadows in the South that seasonally fill with water, alligators commonly build underground passages that link access holes hidden in brush piles. Unless you knew you were in a depression meadow and recognized gator sign (tracks), you could easily have a run-in with one of these rascals. For a very good source on avoiding potentially dangerous animals, pick up a copy of *Survival in the 90s*, by Bob Newman, from Menasha Ridge Press (Birmingham, Alabama).

When you give some thought to all the creatures out there that can ruin your day and maybe your life, it makes sense to always be wary of their whereabouts and take all the necessary steps to avoid having an unpleasant run-in with them. A bear can tear you up; a brown recluse spider can cripple you; a sculptured scorpion can kill you; a rattlesnake can, too; an alligator can grab you and drown you while chewing

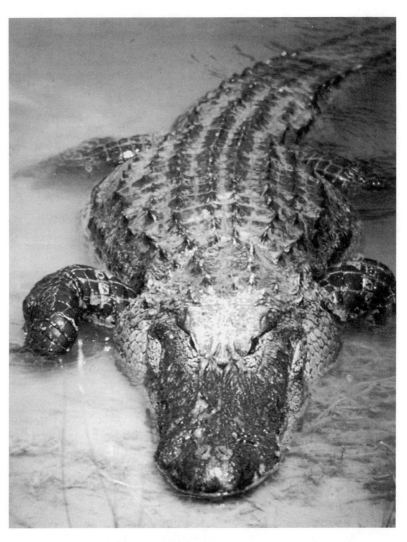

Alligator nests and hides are out of the question.

you up like a baby back rib; a skunk can make you miserable; a porcupine can puncture you; a stingray's barb can hobble you; a man-of-war's sting can set you afire (or so it seems at the time); a catfish can swell your hand to the size of a can-

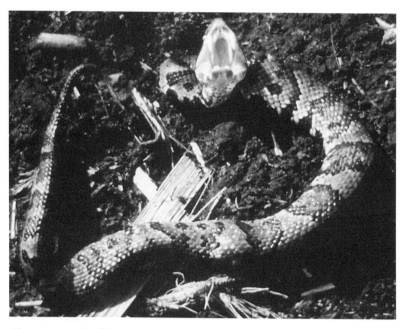

The cottonmouth will put a serious hurt on you.

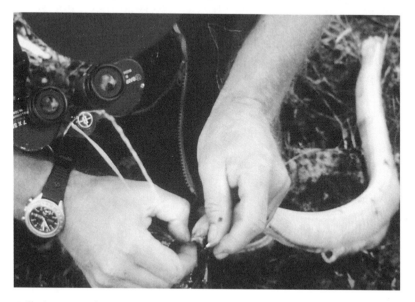

Still, they are good eating.

PRIMITIVE PROSPECTS

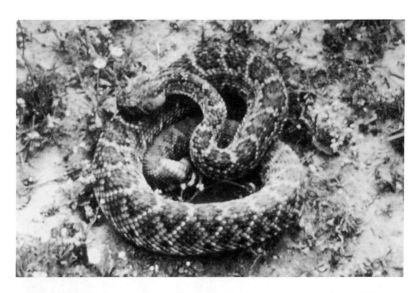

Rattlesnakes come in many sizes and temperaments. (Photo courtesy of U.S. Fish & Wildlife Service)

taloupe; a hive of bees can bring you to your knees; and so on and so on.

All of these problems are nearly always avoidable, although from time to time, no matter what you do to avoid the problem, something is going to get at you.

Attention to detail and a respect for wildlife will set you well on your way to never having a problem with it, whether that wildlife is mammal, insect, arachnid, bird, fish, reptile, crustacean, or what have you. Wishful thinking and complacency are the fugitive's enemy, so watch out for them and keep them out of your camp. I say this from a lot of what is now obviously avoidable experience. Yes, I've been snake-bit, intimidated by bears, growled at by gators, bitten by spiders, stung by bees (and jellyfish and Portugese man-of-wars), and had many other unpleasant interactions with other creatures. Learn from my mistakes, won't you?

ALL THE MAJOR NETWORKS 6

> *"Retch and I arrived at the lake cabin just before dark and went inside and started a fire. Luckily, we were able to smother it before it did much damage."*
>
> —Patrick F. McManus, *Teenagers from Hell*

During World War II in Europe there existed a complicated, very secret organization set up by the Office of Strategic Services (OSS), War Department, intelligence services of other Allied nations, and resistance fighters (loosely known as the *underground*) that conducted clandestine operations against the Nazis. This organization was designed to spirit downed Allied airmen out of Nazi-occupied Europe to safety in Great Britain. It was one of the most effective and daring covert operations of the war, and its foundation remained intact at least into the 1980s in some places as a hedge against war breaking out again in the European theater.

In the century before that war, an equally secret and daring operation run by Harriet Tubman—who was a former slave herself—was used to spirit escaped slaves out of the South to freedom in the North. It was called the *underground railway*, and a great many ex-slaves used it to get to the North with the help of both whites and blacks who all shared a deep-seated hatred for slavery. Many of those who used the underground railway to escape enlisted in the Union Army after war broke out at Fort Sumter, South Carolina, in 1861, to fight against their former owners.

At certain U.S. military schools, evasion networks are set up for students conducting escape and evasion (E&E) training. These networks are manned by military personnel and mature, reliable civilians in the surrounding towns to give the soldiers, sailors, airmen, and Marines the utmost in realism. Many of the civilians who help run the networks are veterans themselves.

During the Gulf War, resistance fighters in Kuwait City were trained to hide downed Coalition pilots and air crews who fell into their hands, and Special Forces (the legendary Green Berets) and Special Air Service (the vaunted British SAS) commandos operating deep inside Iraq were trained to authenticate downed Coalition pilots and extract them from enemy territory.

The U.S. Department of Justice operates an evasion network called the Witness Protection Program, which changes a witness's identity, sets him up with a new life far from his enemies, and then protects him to some degree by maintaining informants who tell them of possible future retaliation against and efforts to locate the witness.

And organized crime continuously operates its own evasion network for those *made guys* who need to disappear for a while or are paying customers. International terrorist organizations have cells in place in various countries that hide terrorists on the run.

All these examples are types of evasion networks, yet you, the real fugitive from whomever and whatever, aren't likely to have it this easy.

THE BAD NEWS

Forget your friends, relatives, and old acquaintances as potential network operators; they are going to be watched and possibly questioned by those looking for you. This means you are going to have to go cold.

Although there have been a great many news accounts of and "investigative reports" on so-called militias recently, only a small percentage of these groups are genuine militias in the traditional sense, which is a group of law-abiding patriots who come to the aid of people in need when the military or police can't lend a hand at the moment, or who take up arms to depose a tyrannical and unacceptably corrupt government. While it's true that most militias are not made up of criminal elements, and most are not plotting the overthrow of the United States, some are no more than bands of ruffians, crooks, con artists, embezzlers, and the like who have joined forces to further feather their own fetid little nests. You can't afford to deal with these people because they will sell you out to the highest bidder at the drop of a hat. Stay clear of them. I would sooner try to buy assistance from the Bloods, Crips, or Hell's Angels than try to use an unfamiliar militia for evasion assistance. And skip the cultish groups like the now mostly dead Branch Davidians, as well as racist extremists; you just can't afford to entrust your freedom to people like this.

On the other hand, you might very well get away with buying assistance from the Mafia, who are generally more reliable and predictable. Still, you risk being exposed by an informant they may not know about. As always, caution is key.

There is no master file of people who are involved in the networks willing to help or hide you. This means that it is going to be up to you to carefully probe for a potential doorman, i.e., the man or woman who will get you into the network, most likely after someone tells them that someone is asking for assistance.

THE GOOD NEWS

There are ways safer than others that will often get you into the network.

If you are in a rural area, especially farm and ranch land in the West, the best place to start may be the church. Approach the local pastor by first speaking to him as he passes a dark area near the rectory or some such place, or be the very last in line for communion during a weekday service and whisper that you must see him after mass in private. (If you are Catholic you can easily contact the priest in the confessional.) Tell him that it is urgent you speak with him in private immediately and assure him that you are harmless and in need of the church's immediate help. Most priests and reverends will take you at your word and bring you into a private office.

Tell the priest that you are in trouble but stress that it is not with the law; have a cover story ready and offer it to him right away. Have a false ID ready. Make your story compelling and believable and ask if there is anyone in his congregation who might be able to hide or otherwise assist you. Continually try to convince him that you are an honest, God-fearing man who is running for his life from some malevolent person or organization seeking to harm or kill you and your family (whom you have spirited away out of the country). The chances are good that the clergyman will make a call and quickly place you with some obscure farmer.

Most farmers and ranchers with large outfits employ hired hands. You should offer to work for room and board (and perhaps a small stipend for miscellaneous expenses) soon after meeting the farmer. This shows him that you are not a freeloader and have a strong work ethic. But be forewarned that farm and ranch life is rigorous; you are going to be working long, hard hours at least six days a week. He is going to be keeping an eye on you, so mind your manners and bust your butt.

Your cover story is going to have to be clean and well-rehearsed, because every hand is going to have to be convinced by the same story *exactly*. Do not drink alcohol or take illegal drugs of any kind. You must live the clean, sober life. Farmers and ranchers—most people in fact—don't take kindly to alcohol or drug abuse, and someone protecting you in the network damn sure won't keep you very long if you demonstrate that you are unstable in any way.

In the city you can also use the church, but city clergymen tend to be more suspicious because of the city environment (i.e., crime and con men are commonplace, and you might fit into that category). Instead, I suggest you visit a bar frequented by longshoremen or other members of a large union. (The most powerful unions have long histories of links to organized crime; in this case, the bad guys are just what you need.) Sit at the bar near the back room (where the extra kegs and other supplies are kept so that when you see the bartender doing some heavy lifting you can lend him a hand) a few nights in a row and make friendly small talk with the barkeep, but don't let on in any way that you need to get into the network or have some kind of problem. Each time you leave the tip should be better than average but not ridiculous. On the fourth or fifth night he'll be calling you by the name you gave him and will consider you more or less a regular.

The next night you come in and appear nervous and concerned. He'll recognize this and ask what's up. Keep up the act and tell him in a conspiratorial tone of voice that you have a big problem and need someone's help—could he direct you to someone who can get you out of sight or out of the area safely for a while?

If he immediately balks, don't pressure him. Instead, get up to leave right away, and as you do so leave him with personal wishes of good luck. For instance, in your small talk with him the nights before he may have mentioned something akin to his son being accepted to Duke. Wish his son the very best as you get up to leave and tell him that it was nice knowing him. Put another above average tip on the bar and walk away. This final act of kindness will sometimes be too much for the guy to take, and he'll stop you and either tell you to sit back down and wait or to go somewhere nearby and wait until contacted.

When your doorman arrives you must do as expected and keep cool. All the same rules apply as in the rural scene. Work for your keep and stay out of trouble.

No matter what network you are in, be cooperative, helpful, and friendly, but never gregarious to a degree that you are doing a lot of talking. The less you say without alienating yourself, the better.

PERSONAL WEAPONS SELECTION 7

"There was a time when the forest was wholly ours and we lived in it as within a fortress. . . . The enemy does not dare to enter."
—William J. Pomeroy
The Huk Guerrilla Struggle in the Philippines

The weapons you select for use during your evasion must be the very best insofar as quality, usefulness, and practicality are concerned. The fugitive cannot afford to make a mistake along these lines. Your weapons can be broken down into two categories: those for hunting and those for defense.

WEAPONS FOR HUNTING

We've already touched briefly on hunting weapons in a general sort of way, but now we need to get into a little more detail so that you make the right choice.

The Rifle

Rifles run the gamut from the itty bitty .17 Remington to monsters like the .577 Nitro Express. This means you have to do some thinking before making your selections.

The .22

Whereas the .22 is fine for squirrels, hares, rabbits, and other species that are small and weak when it comes to getting shot, other species of small game can take a hit from a .22 in what would otherwise be a vital spot and run off on you. In the case of woodchucks, marmots, beavers, muskrats, foxes, and the like, you need something faster, flatter, and more hard-hitting (increased retained muzzle energy), especially if you will be shooting at extended distances. The fugitive can't afford to be shooting game and then having it escape back down its burrow or into the water.

On the other hand, there is a lot to be said for the .22 when it comes to sniping the little guys who are easy prey for the tiny round. If you have the ability to take several firearms with you into your evasion area and there are such little critters available, then take along a reliable .22 such as a Remington Model 541-T, Ruger Model 10/22 (one of the best autoloaders), or a Ruger Model 77/22, which is Ruger's respected and accurate Model 77 downsized into a .22.

Larger Calibers

For those longer shots or for somewhat larger critters like beavers and badgers, a flat-shooting slammer like a .22-250 Remington, .223 Remington (the U.S. military's 5.56mm round like that used in the M16A2 service rifle), .220 Swift, .222 Remington, .222 Remington Magnum, and the like are needed because the .22 just doesn't have the range or the hitting power to fell one of these animals like a round should. Chamber one of these rounds in something like a Winchester Model 70 or Remington Model 700 and you are all set.

Small whitetails, javelina (collared peccary), newborn to yearling deer, caribou, moose, and other such game require a little more oomph. Good calibers include the 6mm Remington, 6.5mm Remington Magnum, .243 Winchester, .257 Roberts,

.25-06 Remington, and the .264 Winchester Magnum, one of my favorites.

The stronger and bigger the game the more important shot placement becomes. You can kill a squirrel with a .22 shot to the midsection with no problem—the thing will die instantly or within a second or two. But when you start dealing with more robust game you are going to have to be more precise. Neck and heart shots are always preferred, with solid (major damage) lung shots also being acceptable. Now you see another reason for having a well-built (read: accurate "out of the box") rifle equipped with an excellent scope. The last thing you want is to be tracking wounded game when evading, and you can't just let the game run off wounded and forget about it because someone who finds that game with a fresh wound will be wondering where you are and may get curious.

Big Rounds

Big whitetails (I don't know, maybe 200 pounds and up?), mule deer, elk, moose, bear, caribou, musk ox, bear, and other hefty critters are considered big game. They call for big, mean rounds like the .300 H&H Magnum, .300 Weatherby Magnum, .300 Winchester Magnum, .338 Winchester Magnum, .340 Weatherby Magnum, and so on. The lowest you should go is a .30-06 Springfield. Avoid monster calibers like the .458 Winchester Magnum—it is just too much and unnecessary.

These big rounds need the very best in a rifle. My personal favorite is a Remington African Plains Rifle chambered in .338 Winchester Magnum. It will take down anything on the continent, and I would even use it in Africa on everything except elephant, rhino, and cape buffalo. Then again, if you are after these last three animals you aren't trying to evade very hard, are you?

The Shotgun

Don't think that you have to be sporting when evading. You don't and shouldn't be. An excellent way to hunt woodchucks and marmots is to lie outside their hole on the upper

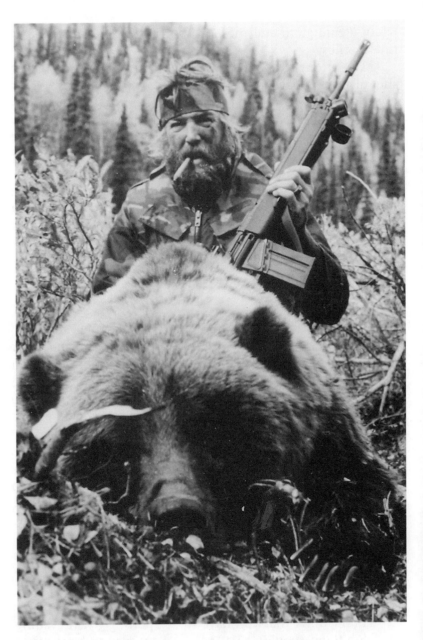

The fugitive must always be ready to defend himself against fellow predators.

ADVANCED FUGITIVE

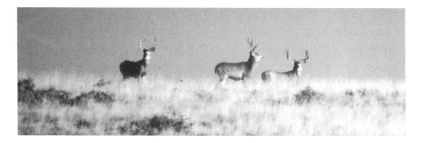

These mule deer bucks demand a big round.

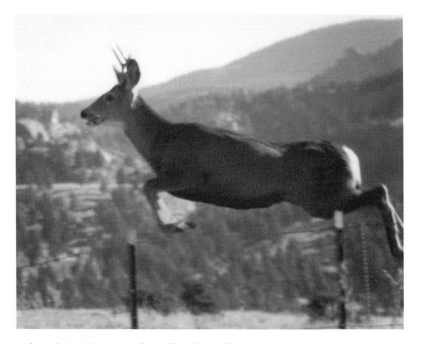

Taking shots at deer doing things like this is seldom advisable.

back side at dawn with a shotgun loaded with No. 4s. These animals are creatures of habit and always come out early in the morning to stretch and eat their breakfast. When they saunter out, shoot them in the head at close range, say, 10 feet or so away from the hole. Don't fire until they are least a few feet from the entrance so they don't fall back in or leap back

PERSONAL WEAPONS SELECTION

down as their final act of defiance. Aside from close ambush of burrowing rodents, the only other time you should be using a shotgun to hunt is when you are firing at flocks of birds on the ground or water, as mentioned earlier. Don't restrict your sluicing to waterfowl, however. Shore birds, turkeys, families of grouse (a hen and her young), and sometimes mammals often gather in groups wherein the individuals are very close to each other. This can be the perfect opportunity to get a lot of food with one shot.

Get a Remington Model 870—a pump gun—in 12 gauge.

The Handgun

Handguns are becoming popular with some hunters. For the fugitive they have limited use and are therefore not for you when it comes to hunting. This is not the case, however, in defense.

WEAPONS FOR DEFENSE

Although the topic of firearms selection for hunting is certainly a broad one, it pales in comparison to firearms selection for defense. The hunting topic can be simplified easily (as I did in the previous section; there's just no need to get into deep, philosophical discussions about weapon designs and ballistics in a book like this), but the principles behind defense call for more thought and discussion.

Rifles

The only rifle you need for self-defense is a high-powered sniper rifle. Now, that said, the debate can be waged until the cows come home about who makes the world's best sniper rifles and what caliber a sniper rifle should be. The point here is that there is no pat answer to these questions except for this: the best sniper rifle/caliber in the world is the weapon that *you* are most effective with. As a caveat to that, however, ballistics and manufacturing techniques do play a critical role in the equation, as does the price of the weapon, i.e., what you can afford. Let's look at all of this.

I spent more than 20 years in a very elite branch of the military (all active duty) and in that branch's most elite community, so I am speaking with no small amount of experience, and yes, bias. But you bought this book for what I have to say on the subject of evasion, so I feel it's appropriate to say here what you paid to hear.

If you look at the sniper rifles used by the military and most SWAT teams in law enforcement organizations, the .308 Winchester (7.62mm) is the caliber of choice. This caliber in a solid rifle with a good scope when match ammo is used is a proven combination, and when you upgrade to a custom-built rifle with a world-class scope and finely tuned, hand-loaded ammunition, you get a beast of a rifle when it is placed in the hands of an expert sniper.

Besides caliber, the rest of the system is broken down into the action, trigger mechanism, barrel, stock (including forearm), and scope. All of these must be made to the most exacting specifications.

The action must be bolt. No action on the whole is more naturally accurate than the bolt. Forget the pump, autoloader, lever, and once-popular falling block; the bolt action is the most solid and gives the best performance when the best of them are placed against one another.

All triggers are not created equal either. Although preferences differ a little from sniper to sniper, a precision-made trigger that can be adjusted with great accuracy is required.

Barrels are a science all unto themselves. Most sniper rifles are made with barrels from the target and varmint genres because they are heavier and have extremely precise lans and grooves. The barrel of your standard deer rifle is nowhere near as accurate as one built for sniping at long ranges.

Most professional (read: they snipe for a living) snipers use custom-fitted fiberglass or fiberglass composite stocks today. Such a stock is easier to care for and adds accuracy to the weapon by being more precisely fitted to the action and barrel and by being as close to flawless in manufacture as you can get—more so than wood can get.

PERSONAL WEAPONS SELECTION

The scope must be special, too, with those made by Unertl being favored by many of the world's best snipers. The Marines use Unertl scopes, which says it all. Second in line is a Svavorski and then a Leupold.

But the best sniper rifle in the world is useless unless it gets into the hands of a good sniper. The fugitive should only use the sniper rifle when he must make a particularly impressive shot on some important game, he is sighting the rifle in (or testing new ammo, a new trigger, or whatever), or he is killing someone coming after him at long range. It shouldn't be your standard varmint rifle.

Handguns

Many volumes have been written about handguns for self-defense, and no doubt many more will be written. Fortunately for the fugitive, this topic can be whittled down to a discussion of caliber and action with a word on sights.

The fugitive needs a handgun chambered in a caliber that gives an outstanding chance of a quick kill with the first well-placed shot. These calibers are 9mm, .44 Magnum, 10mm, .40, and .45 ACP.

By far and away the most popular caliber of handgun used by police and military today is the 9 mil. In the U.S. military the Beretta M9 is standard issue, and it is a decent gun, although not the very best of the best by any stretch of the imagination. In fact, problems with the slide coming detached during firing and striking the operator in the face (with graphic results on one Navy SEAL) had to be addressed and corrected a while back, but it is a good gun nevertheless. However, Sig-Sauer and Glock produce better guns.

The .44 Magnum gained a lot of notoriety as a result of Clint Eastwood's classics *Dirty Harry* and *Magnum Force*, wherein Inspector Harry Callahan toted that big Smith & Wesson Model 29. (Who could forget the diner scene?) The Model 29 is indeed a classic, and it is a good wheel gun if you practice enough with it, but never buy a gun because you saw it used by someone you admire in a movie. Buy a handgun that suits you well instead. If you can handle the recoil of this .44

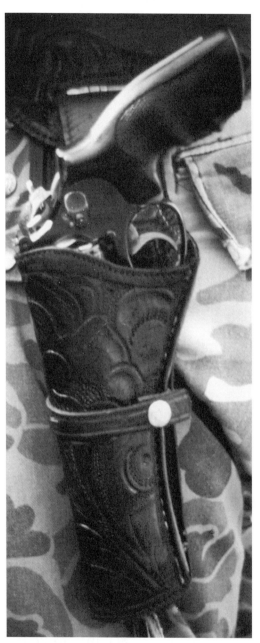

A handgun definitely has a place with the fugitive.

Magnum, then you have a caliber that will certainly do great damage to someone on the first good shot. Wheel guns, though, do have the drawback of only holding six rounds, whereas autoloaders hold several more, sometimes many more.

The 10mm gained attention when the FBI decided that it was the caliber for its agents. It can do a lot of damage in the hands of an expert.

The .45 ACP is my preferred caliber for a handgun. Yes, the old M1911, which was invented by the great gunmaker John Moses Browning in 1898 (it is called the M or Model 1911 because in March of 1911 the U.S. Government accepted Browning's creation as its official sidearm, a position the M1911 held until 1986 when the Beretta M9 replaced it; Colt owned the patent, however), was known for being wildly inaccurate, but the stopping power of the .45 ACP is legendary. The M1911 can be accurized, and many shooters do just that. Glock's .45 ACP is outstanding for accuracy and reliability. (It is interesting to note, however, that Marine special ops units still use a customized version of the M1911 for close-quarters battle or CQB.) An accurized .45 ACP is very hard to beat for killing. *Very* hard.

The fugitive should never be without two handguns on his person, preferably three (a primary gun in a shoulder holster, hip holster, or leg holster, and two backups hidden away). The caliber of each should be the same so that rounds from a gun that goes down (malfunctions) can be loaded into either of the others, and I recommend that the guns are all the same model, too, so that magazines can be interchanged as well.

The gun's sights should be luminous (tritium is best) for firing in dim light. Don't add a scope, but in some cases a laser sight can be very useful.

Shotguns

As a fugitive you need two shotguns. One should be equipped with an extended tubular magazine, and the other should be a sawed-off double-barrel with a pistol grip for those up-close and very personal situations. Twelve gauge is the only gauge, and the action on the primary shotgun should be pump or, failing that, semiautomatic. Pumps are very dependable for the most part (if cared for) and aren't quite as prone to jamming, generally speaking, as the semiauto. Benelli makes some of the best.

The double-barrel (side-by-side) is for the most extreme of emergencies when a very wide pattern is needed at close quarters. Bore the chokes out to skeet.

Shot size is more open to discussion, but I like BB or BBB in my double-barrel (I want a lot of pellets going down range if I am using this gun) and No. 3 buck in my pump. At the ranges in question, BB or BBB in the double gun and No. 3 buck in the pump will do plenty of damage; there is no real need for 00 buck.

Submachine Guns

Yes, it is highly unlikely that you will be evading with a submachine gun unless you are in an elite branch of some military service or have some other special qualifications or experience. Nevertheless, since they are available to some, we need to talk about them.

I am very biased when it comes to submachine guns. Although it's true that there are several very good subguns out there, the one you want (if you have the ability to get what you want) is the H&K MP5A3 or later model. The MP5 series is the most effective, reliable, affordable, and versatile submachine gun in the world. The MAC-10 and Uzi don't even come close.

Knives

There are many different fighting knife designs available. Which is best of all? It's hard to say, but you certainly couldn't go wrong by carrying a Fairbairn-Sykes, the knife made famous for its police use in Shanghai earlier in this century. It worked then and it works today just as well. This double-edged weapon and comparable models (although it could be argued that there *are no* comparable models) can save your butt when everything else goes wrong. Col. Rex Applegate's designs are also very worthy.

Knife fighting is a world of extremes: extreme danger, extreme violence, and extreme adrenalin flow. Given this, the fugitive absolutely must get some training before even beginning to think he is a knife-fighting expert. (This same axiom goes for firearms.) I recommend you start by reading *Street Steel* and then get *Death from the Shadows*, both from Paladin Press.

The fugitive must never be without a knife, just as he must never be without a firearm.

A Word on Hand-to-Hand Combat

Now here's a subject where differences of opinion and controversy thrive.

American interest in hand-to-hand combat exploded with the 1970s television series *Kung Fu* and was bolstered by action movies ("karate flicks") starring the legendary and late

Bruce Lee. The flames were fanned with movies like *The Trial of Billy Jack* and the exploits of such martial arts notables as Bill "Super Foot" Wallace and Chuck Norris. Unfortunately, some people have a difficult time distinguishing between Hollywood and the real world. The fugitive must not.

Hand-to-hand combat where each combatant is fighting for his life rarely involves flying scissor kicks and a blur of nunchaku. Real hand-to-hand combat is usually very sudden, often unexpected, and always ugly, with little thought given to form and style. The last time I fought someone (three months ago as of this writing), the last thing that was going through my mind was how Kwai Chang Cain would have handled the other guy with a quick circle kick and stoic expression. Instead, I was thinking, *How can I knock this asshole out the quickest with the least risk to me?* I had two seconds, as it turned out, to make my decision and the decision I made, when put into action, worked like a charm. (Funny. Even after a career in a very violent world, it takes me nearly an hour to come down from the adrenaline rush of personal combat.)

It is my most sincere recommendation that you avoid forms of self-defense training that stress style and form and karma and inner purity. That stuff is going to get you dead in record time. Instead, save your life by killing the other guy quickly and graphically through the application of extremely aggressive, shockingly violent, and always gruesome personal combat training. The best two in the world are the Marine Corps' LINE (linear in-line neural-override engagement) system and Peyton Quinn's method of adrenaline stress conditioning through scenario-based training (see his book *Real Fighting*). There is also a lot to be said for Gracie family jujitsu, as many of their victims can attest (usually from a bed in intensive care). I am not saying that there is nothing to be gained by gleaning skills from assorted martial arts like kung fu, dim-mak, and the like, because you can learn things in all martial arts that may prove very useful, but spending decades training in one art in which you may never actually *fight* someone is, well, silly.

FIREARMS TRAINING SOURCES

You must choose your firearms training facility with the utmost care. There are many out there that aren't worth your time, effort, or money. The following are recommended.

Gunsite Training Center, Inc.
P.O. Box 700
Paulden, AZ 86334

This is *the* Gunsite, formerly run by Jeff Cooper, one of the world's greatest firearms instructors. A world-class facility with the best of the best instructor staff. Worth every red cent.

Firearms Academy of Seattle, Inc.
P.O. Box 400
Onalaska, WA 98570

For those of you in the Pacific Northwest, this is a solid choice for some excellent training.

Thunder Ranch, Inc.
HCR 1, Box 53
Mountain Home, TX 78058

Nearly on a par with Gunsite.

Yavapai Firearms Academy, Ltd.
P.O. Box 27290
Prescott Valley, AZ 86312

This outfit comes to you and uses local facilities.

SURVIVAL SUPPLY SOURCES

WATER PURIFICATION

General Ecology
151 Sheree Blvd.
Exton, PA 19341

General Ecology makes the world's best portable water filters.

Katadyn USA, Inc.
3020 N. Scottsdale Road
Scottsdale, AZ 85251

Mountain Safety Research (MSR)
4225 2nd Ave. S.
Seattle, WA 98134

PUR
2229 Edgewood Ave. S.
Minneapolis, MN 55426

Sweetwater
2505 Trade Centre Ave.
Longmont, CO 80503

COMPASSES

Brunton USA
620 East Monroe Ave.
Riverton, WY 82501

Silva Compasses
P.O. Box 966
Binghampton, NY 13902

Silva makes the world's best compasses, bar none. Get one of its Rangers.

GLOBAL POSITIONING SYSTEM UNITS

Apelco Marine Electronics
46 River Road
Hudson, NH 03051

Eagle Electronics
P.O. Box 669
Catoosa, OK 74015

Furuno USA, Inc.
271 Harbor Way
South San Francisco, CA 94080

Magellan Systems Corp.
960 Overland Ct.
San Dimas, CA 91773

MAPS

American Education Products
3101 Iris Ave.
Suite 215
Boulder, CO 80301

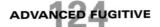

DeLorme Mapping
P.O. Box 298
Freeport, ME 04032

Map Link
25 East Mason St.
Santa Barbara, CA 93101

Trails Illustrated
P.O. Box 4357
Evergreen, CO 80437

FIRST AID EQUIPMENT

Adventure Medical Kits
P.O. Box 43309
Oakland, CA 94624

Dr. Outdoors
P.O. Box 2938
Harlingen, TX 78551

Mountain Medicine USA
Ridge Road
Eaton Center, NH 03832

Sawyer Products
P.O. Box 188
Safety Harbor, FL 34695

Sawyer Products makes the Sawyer Extractor, the best snake bite kit available. Get one.

Wisconsin Pharmacal
P.O. Box 198
Jackson, WI 53037

GENERAL SUPPLIERS

L.L. Bean
Casco St.
Freeport, ME 04032

The emperor of outdoor gear, L.L. Bean offers a lifetime guarantee on everything it sells, no questions asked. One of a kind. Its store in Freeport is a holy place.

FIREARMS ACCESSORY SUPPLY SOURCES

Delta Force
P.O. Box 1625
El Dorado, AR 71731

Kramer Handgun Leather, Inc.
P.O. Box 112154
Tacoma, WA 98411

Law Concealment Systems, Inc.
P.O. Box 3952
Wilmington, NC 28406

Matthews Police Supply Co.
P.O. Box 1754
Matthews, NC 28105

Michigan Body Armor
P.O. Box 251423
West Bloomfield, MI 48325

Moore Technical Industries
P.O. Box 1705
Cottonwood, AZ 86326

USA Magazines, Inc.
P.O. Box 39115
Downey, CA 90239

SOURCES FOR SURVEILLANCE AND COUNTERSURVEILLANCE DEVICES

A.M.C. Sales, Inc.
193 Vaquero Dr.
Boulder, CO 80303

Excalibur Enterprises
P.O. Box 400
Fogelsville, PA 18051-0400

Executive Protection Products, Inc.
1325 Imola Ave. W.
Suite S
Napa, CA 94559

First Witness Video Surveillance Systems
300 N. Central Ave.
Staunton, VA 24401

Morovision
219 Broadway
Suite 307
Laguna Beach, CA 92651

Silver Creek Industries
P.O. Box 1988
Manitowoc, WI 54221

Spy Outlet
P.O. Box 337
Buffalo, NY 14226

Visiontek Night Vision
1200 Industrial Road #17
San Carlos, CA 94070

CAMOUFLAGE CLOTHING SOURCES

Advantage
P.O. Box 9638
Columbus, GA 31908-9101

Backland
6053 Hudson Road
Suite 280
Woodbury, MN 55125

Brigade Quartermasters
1025 Cobb Int. Blvd.
Kennesaw, GA 30144-4300

Bushlan Camouflage
313 Mill Run
Kerrville, TX 78028

Cabela's
812 13th Ave.
Sidney, NE 69160

Columbia Sportswear
P.O. Box 83239
Portland, OR 97283-0239

Day One Camouflage
3300 S. Knox Ct.
Denver, CO 80110

Haas Outdoors
P.O. Box 757
West Point, MS 39773

Ideal Products
101 W. DuBois Ave.
DuBois, PA 15801

Kelly Cooper
P.O. Box 49
Picture Rocks, PA 17762

Natgear
4209 S. Shackleford
Suite D
Little Rock, AR 72204

Photo Stealth
111 Dennis Dr.
Lexington, KY 40503

Predator
2605 Coulee Ave.
La Crosse, WI 54601

Shannon Outdoors
Rt. 3, Box 77
Winnsboro, SC 29180

Skyline
184 Ellicott Rd.
West Falls, NY 14170

Spartan/Realtree
P.O. Box 9638
Columbus, GA 31908-9638

Sticks N' Limbs/Freddie
Bear Sports
17250 Oak Park Ave.
Tinely Park, IL 60477

Timber Ghost
10022 CR 3070
Rolla, MO 65401

Trebark
3434 Buck Mountain Rd.
Roanoke, VA 24014

Trevanish
2169 Greenville Road
LaGrange, GA 30240

SURVIVAL TRAINING SOURCES

Exercise extreme caution when selecting a survival training school or course. There are several out there that are staffed and taught by unqualified personnel, or that stress holistic, New Age crap. Fugitives don't need that trash. There are only two schools I would recommend that are in some way useful to the fugitive.

National Outdoor Leadership School (NOLS)
288 Main Street
Lander, WY 82520

NOLS has outstanding instructors and offers various courses in outdoor skills.

World Survival Institute (WSI)
P.O. Box 394C
Tok, AK 99780

Run by Chris Janowsky, author of *Survival: A Manual that Could Save Your Life* (Paladin Press), WSI is the leading hard-core survival school in the country.

RECOMMENDED READING

Angier, Bradford. *Field Guide to Edible Wild Plants*. Harrisburg: Stackpole, 1974. Bradford Angier has been called "the dean of American survivalists." The term is accurate.

Craighead, Frank C., and John J. Craighead Jr. *How to Survive on Land and Sea*. Annapolis: Naval Institute Press, 1943. An outstanding book that is used in the Department of Defense Survival School System.

Foster, Steven, and Roger Caras. *Venomous Animals and Poisonous Plants*. Boston: Houghton Mifflin, 1994.

Gill, Paul G. Jr., M.D. *Simon & Schuster's Pocket Guide to Wilderness Medicine*. New York: Simon & Schuster, 1991.

Isaac, Jeff, P.A.C., and Peter Goth, M.D. *The Outward Bound Wilderness First Aid Handbook*. New York: Lyons & Burford, 1991.

Janowsky, Chris. *Survival*. Boulder, CO: Paladin Press, 1986. Chris Janowsky runs the World Survival Institute in Tok, Alaska, and is a frequent contributor to *American Survival Guide*.

Krochmal, Arnold, and Connie Krochmal. *A Field Guide To Medicinal Plants*. New York: Times, 1973.

Newman, Bob. *Wilderness Wayfinding*. Boulder, CO: Paladin Press, 1994. This superior land navigation and survival book is used as a reference at the Navy Survival School in Maine, where the author taught for a few years. Bob Newman is the author of several excellent books on survival-related topics and the host of an outstanding educational video, *The Ultimate Outdoorsman* (Paladin Press).

Shanks, Bernard. *Wilderness Survival*. New York: Universe, 1980. Bernard Shanks is one of the world's most respected survivalists.

ABOUT THE AUTHOR

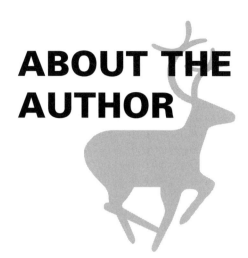

Kenn Abaygo has written numerous books and many hundreds of magazine articles and newspaper columns. His work has appeared in some of the most popular outdoor skill-related publications in the United States.

Formally and thoroughly trained in evasion during his more than 20 years of federal employment, during which time he taught evasion and survival skills to selected personnel, Kenn Abaygo's first evasion book, *Fugitive: How to Run, Hide, and Survive,* is one of Paladin's best-selling survival manuals. He took his pseudonym from Kennebago Lake in western Maine, where he enjoys fly fishing for trout and salmon.

He is currently involved in the filming of a video based on the *Fugitive* series, to be released by Paladin Press.